Human–Computer Interaction Series

SpringerBriefs in Human-Computer Interaction

Series editors

Desney Tan, Microsoft Research, USA
Jean Vanderdonckt, Université catholique de Louvain, Belgium

More information about this series at http://www.springer.com/series/15580

Alberto Del Bimbo · Andrea Ferracani
Daniele Pezzatini · Lorenzo Seidenari

Natural Interaction in Medical Training

Tools and Applications

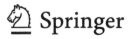 Springer

Alberto Del Bimbo
Faculty of Engineering
University of Florence
Florence
Italy

Andrea Ferracani
Media Integration and Communication
    Center
University of Florence
Florence
Italy

Daniele Pezzatini
Media Integration and Communication
    Center
University of Florence
Florence
Italy

Lorenzo Seidenari
Media Integration and Communication
    Center
University of Florence
Florence
Italy

ISSN 1571-5035
Human–Computer Interaction Series
ISSN 2520-1670   ISSN 2520-1689   (electronic)
SpringerBriefs in Human-Computer Interaction
ISBN 978-3-319-61035-1   ISBN 978-3-319-61036-8   (eBook)
https://doi.org/10.1007/978-3-319-61036-8

Library of Congress Control Number: 2017958630

Printed on acid-free paper

This Springer imprint is published by Springer Nature
The registered company is Springer International Publishing AG
The registered company address is: Gewerbestrasse 11, 6330 Cham, Switzerland

Contents

Chapter 1
Introduction

Abstract In the last decades, there has been a significant increase in the adoption of simulation systems in the medical field. More attention to patient safety, combined with the need to reserve more hours to operators for efficient individual and team training, has opened the way to the adoption of new technologies and innovative processes. This progress is happening also borrowing examples and principles from professions that have established training programs such as the military or the aviation. In particular, this book discusses motivations and opportunities offered by recent advances in information technology that can be exploited in this field and review a robust literature that is continuously growing up. The main objective is to show how trending technologies such as virtual reality, natural interaction, and applied computer vision can be used in an integrated way to improve traditional training systems (Part of this chapter previously appeared in Ferracani et al. (Proceedings of the 2014 ACM international workshop on serious games. ACM Inc., pp 27–32, 2014 [1]) © 2014 Association for Computing Machinery, Inc. Reprinted by permission; and in Ferracani et al. (Univ Access Inf Soc 14(3):351–362, 2015 [2]) with permission of Springer.).

Keywords Medical simulation · Technology · Applications

1.1 Book Overview

Simulation and training for medical personnel is of paramount importance in order to achieve high success rate in emergency and stressful situations. Many kinds of simulations exist, from simple point-and-click serious games to expensive mannequins, instrumented and animated to deliver realistic symptoms for medical conditions and induce adequate responses from healthcare professionals. Medical simulation is covered by existing manuals and by a wide literature; nonetheless in this short book, we offer a unique point of view combining know-how and experiences from medical professionals and computer engineers focused on immersive and natural interaction techniques. The use of 3D in computer applications can increase the sense of immersion of the operators and therefore improve the veracity of the simulation. Immersive 3D visualization technologies (such as low-cost head-mounted displays or CAVEs)

© The Author(s) 2017   1
A. Del Bimbo et al., *Natural Interaction in Medical
Training*, SpringerBriefs in Human-Computer Interaction,
https://doi.org/10.1007/978-3-319-61036-8_1

are commercially available, and there has been a lot of research on the interaction methods that can be provided to a user moving and acting through virtual 3D environments. These interaction methods aim to capture human gestures and voice input to control the simulation. Recent progress in real-time vision-based approaches for understanding gestures and interactions can effectively bridge the gap in natural communication between humans and computer interfaces. In particular, we are going to discuss methods for natural interaction which provide virtual reality environments with (1) action and voice recognition; and (2) re-identification capabilities. We are also going to explain why these two 'features' are important and to propose technologies and new approaches for maximizing human–computer interaction through efficient recognition systems satisfying real-time requirements. In order to do this, we will present two prototype systems which exploit these technologies: a Basic Life Support and Defibrillation system and a Surgical Safety Checklist system which both use natural interaction and virtual reality for healthcare professionals training. Evaluation results show how the adoption of 'natural interaction' techniques can lead to a significant improvement of the simulation experience and trainees' learning.

1.1.1 Case Studies

In Chap. 4, we are going to present and assess evaluation results (through quantitative and qualitative studies) of the two prototypes we developed, i.e., the Basic Life Support and Defibrillation (BLSD-S) and the Surgical Safety Checklist (SSC-S) simulators which are the main subject of this book.

BLSD-S: This prototype allows simulation and training of medical and paramedical personnel in an emergency medicine scenario. Immersive simulations in emergency situations are extremely useful to confront operators with scenarios that can also be extreme (e.g., a car accident with several injured people) without posing the simulation participants in any harm. The prototype allows operators to simulate an immersive scenario of a gas leak in a house with an unconscious person on the floor. This person has to be re-animated following the correct procedure. Trainees can interact using gestures to move in the room, secure the environment, and assist the patient. Natural interaction (locomotion and gestures) is provided in two different ways that we compare in two different versions of the simulator, i.e., BLSD-S (I) and BLSD-S (II), which exploit different depth sensors for interaction detection: (1) the Microsoft Kinect™ sensor and (2) the Leap Motion sensor. The main difference between the use of these two devices is that their different capabilities have inspired and allowed the design and implementation of diverse interaction modalities. These capabilities have also affected which medical procedures can be simulated and at what extent can be performed with completely natural gestures. The Microsoft Kinect ™ sensor is deployed in a scenario where the user stands in the room in front of the sensor and the simulation is projected on a big wall (since the Kinect can track all the body figure), while the Leap Motion allows the user to interact with the virtual simulation sitting on the chair and wearing a head-mounted display (despite the fact that the Leap Motion allows to track only the user hands, it gives accurate information on fingers positions that can be exploited to efficiently carry out the simulation).

SSC-S: Although many medical simulators exist with the aim to train personal skills of medical operators, only few of them take into account cooperation between team members. After the introduction of the Surgical Safety Checklist by the World Health Organization (WHO) that has to be carried out by surgical team members before an operation and that is constituted by a list of procedures intended to ensure safe surgery and minimize complications, several studies have proved that the adoption of this procedure can remarkably reduce the risk of a surgical crisis. The SSC-S prototype exposes a natural interface featuring an interactive virtual environment that aims to train medical professionals in following the WHO security procedures. The interface adopts a 'serious game' approach. The system presents a realistic and immersive 3D interface (projected on the wall) and allows multiple users to interact using vocal input and hand gestures. Natural interactions between users and the simulator are provided exploiting the Microsoft Kinect™ sensor. The interface follows the paradigms of a role play game in which every trainee has to perform the correct procedure steps of the checklist accordingly to his professional role in the medical team (i.e., the anesthesiologist, the surgeon or the nurse).

1.2   Who This Book Is For

This book is aimed at practitioners, researchers, hospitals, and medical institutions managers who want to have insights into state-of-the-art techniques and possible solutions in the use of medical-related technologies for training. Training of students and operators in medical procedures can really benefit from the adoption of the technologies presented that have been proved effective in minimizing medical errors in real scenarios in comparison with standard procedures. The book is also for experienced human–computer interaction engineers working with medical staff, but also with experts and professionals in other domains, who want to deepen some innovative and possible approaches in leveraging computer vision and natural interaction technologies in immersive training environments.

Acknowledgements The two simulation prototypes presented in this book have been developed in the context of the project RIMSI Integrated Research of Simulation Models for the validation of processes and prototypes in surgical and emergency medicine, funded by Regione Toscana, Italy.

References

1. Ferracani A, Pezzatini D, Bimbo A D (2014) A natural and immersive virtual interface for the surgical safety checklist training. In Proceedings of the 2014 ACM international workshop on serious games. ACM Inc., pp 27–32. https://doi.org/10.1145/2656719.2656725
2. Ferracani A, Pezzatini D, Seidenari L, Bimbo A D (2015) Natural and virtual environments for the training of emergency medicine personnel. Univ Access Inf Soc, 14(3), pp 351–362. Springer

Chapter 2
Natural Interaction for Medical Simulation and Training

Abstract Skills training is of primary importance for healthcare professionals. New technologies such as natural interfaces and virtual reality bring new possibilities in learning outcomes especially if used synergically exploiting some principles derived from the so-called serious gaming interfaces. Virtual reality combined with natural interaction interfaces, through which natural gestures can be used to control interaction, have been primarily used in the medical field for the development of rehabilitation systems. However, such technologies are also promising for the implementation of decision support and skill training systems since they can improve users engagement in task completion and team based activities through immersivity and physical participation. In this chapter we are going to give an overview of the current state of medical simulation, considering issues and new perspectives, and to explain why immersive digital systems and natural interaction are important and can contribute to improving medical training. A large literature on immersive and natural interaction systems is reviewed highlighting good practices and limits. New opportunities offered by the recent development of virtual reality, especially if combined with computer vision systems, are introduced.

Keywords Natural interaction · Immersive environments · Virtual reality

2.1 Introduction

Medical simulations have been enacted for centuries, even in primitive forms [1]. Practice is a key component for the maintenance and learning of skills in medicine [2], and in this regard, medical simulation encompasses different solutions. According to the pioneer David Gaba [3], there are five categories of simulation in medicine: verbal simulations, standardized patients, part-task trainers, electronic patients, and computer patients. A verbal simulation is a role-playing game between trainees. Standardized patients are actors employed to train junior doctors in communication and physical examination skills as well as patient history taking. Task trainers usually are lifelike models of body parts, such as an arm or pelvis, and the most complex versions are also used as surgical trainers, use mechanics, and can be useful

© The Author(s) 2017
A. Del Bimbo et al., *Natural Interaction in Medical Training*, SpringerBriefs in Human-Computer Interaction,
https://doi.org/10.1007/978-3-319-61036-8_2

in teaching biological processes. Electronic patients are probably the most realistic devices for simulations. They are full-size heavy mannequins[1] with human-like behavior (e.g., providing eye blinking, breathe, and pulse) and are usually computer controlled in order to induce disease symptoms. Electronic patients and dedicated electronic devices such as task trainers allow to carry out rather plausible simulations. Compared to standardized patients and verbal simulations, they can return symptoms and body reactions not otherwise reproducible in a feasible and realistic way using actors. They also allow to repeat simulations as often as it is needed without additional staff costs. On the other hand, these simulators are very expensive and not easily sustainable with regard to maintenance costs. Computer patients, especially if exploiting VR and natural interaction, can be used to reduce this cost: in fact they can provide virtual software based interactive characters capable of giving the same visual, auditory and sensory feedback of standardized and electronic patients with an acceptable degree of realism at a much lower overall and maintenance cost.

Simulation in medical training has really improved in both fidelity and performance, though there are still several issues that entail an in some cases justified skepticism in its adoption during the training process. Nonetheless, several schools of medicine all around the world are integrating simulations in doctor training and even offer certifications recognized by simulation centers [4]. The main reason of the delay in this adoption is related to several factors such as the cost of professional training personnel and the cost of the equipment and its maintenance (e.g., for the purchase and maintenance of electronic mannequins for patients simulations or the use of special devices for interaction such as motors and haptic controllers). These problems can be largely mitigated through the adoption of computer patients exploiting latest technological progresses in natural interaction (NI), 3D computer graphics, and VR applied to simulations. In fact, new paradigms of interaction and improvements in the realism of virtual environments can now inspire to engineers and professionals the design of software-based learning tools for activities training ranging from medium to high complexity, also in the medical field. In this book, we give some suggestions on how to exploit advanced techniques such as natural interaction and computer vision applied to two VR scenarios pointing out also the limits that these technologies may present in other scenarios.

However, despite some limitations we are going to explain in the rest of the book, it is evident that natural and VR interfaces can reduce the cost of simulation replacing expensive infrastructures, interaction controllers, and necessary medical equipment devices with virtual worlds. Moreover, simulation of dangerous and extreme scenarios can be carried out without risk and with a higher level of contextual awareness and engagement provided by high-fidelity realistic rendering and natural interaction paradigms and techniques boosted by computer vision. In this way, the quality of the training of junior and professional personnel can be really improved. In particular, compared to simulations with mannequins, these computer systems allow to:

---

[1] 'Harvey mannequin' was one of the earliest electronic patients, currently sold by Laerdal Corporation.

- have an intelligent and configurable system that responds automatically to user actions;
- receive continuous audiovisual feedback from the ambient;
- simulate situations similar to those recreated with the use of mannequins, but at a lower cost, enhancing the realism of environments, of the interaction and of the communication through VR and NI. Consequently, this improves learnability and memorability of procedures;
- be corrected on the fly and have human-like system feedback in real time. Feedback is usually provided in the debriefing phase in standard medical training. In this part of the training, trainers and trainees discuss the simulation sessions. This approach assumes a period of time between the wrong action and the correction which instead is provided simultaneously during the computer-based simulation.

However, the effective gain in using these computer systems featuring VR and especially NI also depends on the simulation objectives. In fact, medical simulation systems can have different goals such as training communication between members of a team, providing situational awareness and teaching procedures, exercising on manual skills. Skills training in particular requires precise measurements and high-level human evaluation of procedures accomplishments. In these situations, a few millimeters of error may result in a critical outcome for the patient as in the case of a surgical operation. On the other hand, it is really difficult to obtain granular and effective virtual simulation for personal skill training using, for example, natural interaction (that it is not so accurate for understanding the movements of a surgeon's hands during e.g., a laparoscopy), while for improving intra-team members communication and situational awareness using the same technologies, there is usually the need of supporting a sufficient complexity in the scenario. In this latter case, there could be a proportionally growing difficulty in scenario understanding which, conversely, is an essential prerequisite for the adoption of NI and computer vision in VR simulators. For example, while assisting a pediatric patient, parents may interfere with the procedure, though at the same time they are probably the only and most accurate source of information on the patient's history and the cause of his/her condition. It can be quite challenging to reproduce this virtual scenario in an immersive environment and simultaneously to allow all these actors be enacted by trainees capable of interacting naturally with the VR interface. These are important points that have to be taken into account when considering the adoption of natural interaction applied to virtual environments for training. The two prototypes we are going to present in this book in Chap. 4 make use of these technologies but previous in-depth studies on usability and systems objectives as well as on the interaction design of simulations have been conducted in order to asses the effectiveness of these technologies in those scenarios with respect to the objectives and to ensure the feasibility of the final simulators. In fact, natural interaction, at the state of the art, is not so mature to be exploited in scenarios which require continuous high-fidelity gesture tracking and a high-level understanding of a complex situation. Furthermore, also when NI can be adopted, it may need adaptations to the context of use and the introduction of new design strategies as those we explain for the SSC-S simulator presented in Sect. 4.3.

It is, however, indisputable that computer simulation systems (also those not exploiting advanced features such as Virtual Reality and Natural Interaction which add realism and engagement with the systems) can offer great benefits with regard to the management and the cost of professional training. This is a point that should be stressed considering several aspects. For example, to improve medical operators' communication skills it is also important to be able to repeat simulations. Simulations may be repeated with the same configuration parameters or with slight variations. This kind of simulation and configuration is usually performed working on expensive electronic patients or mannequins under the supervision of professionals. Furthermore, instrumentation and configuration of the parameters have to be controlled in loco by instructors, impacting heavily on staff costs. McIntosh et al. [5] have analyzed the expenses related to 'classic' training systems of several simulation centers in a 2006 article. Results showed that the overall set-up cost for facilities and equipment was $876,485. Fixed costs per year amounted at a total of $361,425, while variable costs for session training and teaching totaled $311 per course hour.

Simulation scenarios in which such systems can prove to be highly suitable and convenient can certainly be found in the field of emergency medicine training where they can be extremely useful to teach emergency medical technicians (EMTs) and medics to operate in harmful or critical situations. In fact, the use of computer simulators allows reproducing the environment of also extreme scenarios in a more realistic way (e.g., a plane crash or an earthquake). In fact, the use of computer simulators allows to reproduce the environment of also extreme scenarios in a realistic way (e.g., a plane crash or an earthquake). However, it should be said that for some aspects, as when an operator has to interact with the patient, virtual environments may also be poor in returning the realism of the simulation with respect to electronic patients, since it would be complicated, for example, to deliver the tactile information that a physical electronic mannequin, or a real human, can. Despite these considerations, VR is an essential way of reducing training costs while maintaining at the same time good performance in skill acquisition, even more valuable in the future if we consider its integration with NI interfaces, which is one of the subject of this book, and the fact that multimedia systems are more and more capable of providing realistic and multisensory feedback. Furthermore, through computer simulators (1) environmental conditions can be easily varied so to reinforce environmental awareness in the trainees; (2) number of patients in need of assistance and operators can be increased in the simulation with no cost at all especially if they are non-playing characters (NPC). As an example, let us imagine the scenario of a bus crash on a highway. Such a scenario requires the intervention of multiple medical operators with a high skill in managing and prioritizing patient assistance procedures. The enactment of such a simulation scenario would require a vast amount of free ground, several electronic patients, and actors together with trainees. Electronic mannequins are quite expensive since their cost ranges from 20k to 80k $. Only a few medical schools and the military can afford such expenses. Therefore, simulations involving the use of electronic mannequins are usually enacted in the emergency room or in a bare room at the hospital with an availability of only one or two electronic patients. Furthermore, the possibility for operators to be confronted with situations involving many risks both for the patient and themselves can improve the trainees environmental awareness and the interrelational skills of the operators. These situations and the actual actions to be performed can be simulated realistically not only at no cost but without any risk for the trainees. An example is a Basic Life Support and Defibrillation (BLSD) scenario in an apartment of a burning building where simulation participants need to take care of their safety before assisting the patient requesting, if needed, firemen support (the same scenario is provided in description of our BLSD-S simulator in Sect. 4.2.2).

Dale [6] has carried out a comparative evaluation of methods of information delivery in education. On this basis, he has proposed his famous 'cone of experience' which highlights how higher learning outcomes are achieved when concepts are delivered in a form that is as close as possible to the real experience. Therefore, taking part in a realistic VR simulation which provides high quality graphics rather than trying to imagine a situation or worse passively watching videos or reading can increase the amount of information that can be effectively memorized by a student. Medical education can really benefit from new technologies providing immersive and natural interfaces which can allow trainers to teach and debrief well-defined procedures, as well as learners to acquire a high level of participation and control. Nowadays, this can be achieved through several types of solutions that allow different levels of perceptual and psychological immersion: 3D graphics visualized on standard displays, specialized rooms (e.g., Cave), or VR exploited through head-mounted displays (HMDs) together with interaction devices for the 3D world (e.g., Kinect, Razer Hydra, force feedback gloves, haptic devices).

In the following sections, we review and discuss different types of medical simulation systems, ranging from simple desktop applications to highly interactive virtual reality (VR) simulators. We are also going to introduce the concept of natural interaction and his application to the medical field. A summary of the presented simulations systems discussed in this chapter can be found in Table 2.1.

2.2 Applications for Medical Simulation and Training

2.2.1 Medical Simulation Systems

The literature in the field of medical training systems reveals, in recent years, an orientation toward the design of high configurable prototypes [3, 7–9]. These systems are difficult to implement and maintain due to the fact that medical procedures are becoming everyday more complex. On the other hand, very specialized systems [10, 11] have been designed in a way that makes them not adaptable and flexible enough to be deployed in different scenarios. Furthermore, for the most part, the majority of interfaces of these systems are not fully immersive and intuitive. Nonetheless, although they exploit different tools for interaction such as haptic sensors, cameras, and markers, they could benefit a lot from natural interaction techniques.

The Cybermed framework [7] is a system for medical training via computer network. It has advanced features for configuring some aspects of the simulation such as the number of users, the gestures to manipulate the objects, the type of devices (mouse or haptic systems) to be exploited, and the choice of the actors for remote mentoring and distance learning (tutor or participants) but it does not really allow an exhaustive characterization of the situation or the definition of complex medical procedures. SOFA [8], ViMet [9], and GiPSi [12] frameworks instead are open-source projects which feature a high level of modularity and rely on the capability of a multi-model representation of simulation models (deformable models, collision models, instruments).

Although they easily allow to simulate a scenario, say a laparoscopy, they neither provide a real natural and immersive interface nor they go beyond enabling the system to respond to punctual stimuli (e.g., in the laparoscopy use case, deformation of the liver, and collision with the ribs). Spring [10] is a more specific mouse-based desktop framework for real-time surgical simulations which provides a basic configurability for patient-specific anatomy. Laerdal MicroSim [11] is a non-immersive simulation system that presents to trainees pre-hospital, in-hospital, and military scenarios. In the pre-hospital scenario, the user can interact with the patient through a simple 2D interface and has a static view of the scene. Recent studies [13, 14] instead have proved the benefits of the use of game dynamics to boost the adoption of simple computer-based virtual patients by groups of students for medical training sessions.

With regard to more immersive solutions, Honey et al. have created a virtual environment in second life for hemorrhage management [15]; Cowan et al. [16] have developed a system for the inter-professional education (IPE) for critical care providers where an immersive 3D situation is accessed across the network in a 'multi-player online' environment, allowing trainees to participate, as avatars, from remote locations. Sliney et al. [17] propose a system, named JDoc, which uses realistic situations to train junior doctors in dealing with the frenzy of a first aid hospital. Immersivity and realism are one of the keypoints for users engagement in the development of these training systems. This is confirmed by Buttussi et al. [18] who obtained encouraging results evaluating a 3D serious game as a support tool for medicine students.

2.2.2 Immersive Interactive Environments (IVEs) and Serious Gaming

The concept of 'serious games' has been used since the 1960s whenever referring to solutions adopting gaming with educational purpose rather than pure players' entertainment [19]. Among the different fields of study in which serious games have been exploited, medicine is one the most prolific [20] counting a large number of applications that feature immersive virtual environments (IVEs). Improvements in medical training using gaming and IVEs have been brought out especially in the field of surgical education where IVEs already play a significant role in training programs [21, 22].

The Off-Pump Coronary Artery Bypass (OPCAB) game [23] and the Total Knee Arthroplasty game [24], for example, focus on the training of decision-taking dynamics in a virtual operating room. Serious games featuring IVEs about different topics are Pulse! [25], for acute care and critical care, CAVE™triage training [26], or Burn Center™ for the treatment of burn injuries [27]. Though all these medical training simulators focus on individual skills, an important aspect of health care to be taken into account is that, for the most, it has to be provided by teams. Common techniques of team training in hospitals include apprenticeship, role playing, and rehearsal and involve high costs due to the required personnel, simulated scenarios that often lack realism, and the large amount of time needed. Several serious games featuring IVEs for team training have also been developed in the last years. 3DiTeams [25], CliniSpace™[28], HumanSim [29], Virtual ED [30], and Virtual ED II [31] are some examples of gaming approaches in team training for acute and critical care whose main objective is to identify and reduce the weaknesses in operational procedures. A virtual environment for training combat medics has been developed by Wiederhold and Wiederhold [32] to prevent the eventuality of post-traumatic stress disorder. Medical team training for emergency first response has been developed as systems distributed over the network by Alverson et al. [33] and Kaufman et al. [34].

IVEs have proved to be an effective educational tool. Tasks can be repeated in a safe environment and as often as required. IVEs, as we have stressed in the previous section, allow to realistically experience a wide range of situations that would be impossible to replicate in the real world due to danger, complexity, and impracticability. Though IVEs have been traditionally associated with high costs due to the necessary hardware, especially to provide real-time interactivity (multiple projectors, input devices, etc.), and have always presented a difficult setup, in the last years these issues have been partially solved by the availability of cheap and easily deployable devices such as head-mounted displays (e.g., the Oculus Rift, the Samsung Gear VR) for VR and controllers or depth sensors (e.g., the Nintendo Wii or the Microsoft Kinect™) for providing interaction, context understanding, or reconstruction. A realistic representation of the environment and the naturalness of interaction, made possible by these devices, allows to create in learners the correct mental model and to reinforce the memorability of specific procedures. On the basis of the constructivism theory [35], one of the main features of educational IVEs is the possibility of providing highly interactive experiences capable to intellectually engage trainees in carrying out tasks and activities they are responsible for. The opportunity to navigate educational scenarios as first person controllers (especially through HMD) allows learners to have a more direct awareness of the interaction context and of their responsibilities than in sessions mediated through an un-related element such as a graphical user interface or an other symbolic representation. In this regard, IVEs present a less cognitive effort in elaborating the context and stimulate imagination. This is even more true in scenarios where not only skills are learned in the environment where these will be applied, but also the tasks can be carried out by the trainee acting in a natural way without the mediation of any device (e.g., keyboard, mouse, or other controllers). It is also pointed out by constructivists that learning is enhanced when gaming, group-work activity, and cooperation are provided. Interacting with humans is more interesting and involving than interacting with a computer, and it implies personal responsibility. Each learner is expected by others to account for his/her actions and to contribute to the achievement of the team goal. The use of gaming techniques in education is called 'edutainment,' and it is preferred by trainees to the traditional approaches because it increases students motivation and engagement in the learning context [36].

Despite the perceived advantages and the good appreciation of serious games featuring IVEs for training, the adoption of such systems is still poor in real medical facilities. This is due to the fact that some open issues still exist in the usability of systems exploiting latest technologies in NI and VR. For example: (1) NI provides poor accuracy in detecting complex gestures; (2) some open problems exist on how to move naturally in virtual spaces being constrained in physical spaces; (3) it is easy to get lost in VR due to the possibility of free movement; it is difficult to provide a significant set of options in VR environments without switching to traditional device-controlled 2D interfaces (e.g., panels visualizing multiple choices or drop-down menus). Things are even more complicated when we talk about multi-user systems for team training. Eventually, we can say that well-designed VR systems could benefit a lot adopting natural interaction techniques and exploiting new low-cost devices available on the market for navigating and controlling interfaces provided that the limitations of the technologies themselves are taken into account and interfaces are designed accordingly. In Chap. 3, we show how some techniques of computer vision applied to NI can improve the capabilities of these systems.

2.3   Natural Interaction Applications

2.3.1   Interaction Techniques and Devices

The basic idea of natural interaction (NI) is to create a more intuitive and natural human–computer communication, inspired by real-life interactions such as speech, gestures, and touch. The mutual progress in the field of human–computer interaction, computer vision, and pattern recognition has made possible to propose such technologies for providing natural gestures to control digital interfaces. Systems adopting natural interaction show increased efficiency, speed, power, and realism in many fields. Medical simulation systems, and educational application in general, can also benefit from the adoption of NI. Several Natural User Interfaces (NUIs) featuring natural interaction systems have been used in medical rehabilitation, although sparsely, leveraging different technologies (e.g., Nintendo Wii, PlayStation EyeToy), as part of physical therapy. Haptic sensors are commonly used in rehabilitation to ease the interaction with the systems [37, 38]. Markers and accelerometers/gyroscopes provided by the Nintendo Wii have been used to get information about scene orientation and objects positioning in order to augment and improve systems responsiveness [39] to human behaviors. These solutions, despite being easy to implement, have the disadvantage to be not completely natural, forcing users to wear or to hold different devices with their hands in order to interact with the systems [40]. A more natural way to interact is commonly obtained allowing user to perform gestures with their hands in an unobtrusive way. Early adopter of gesture-based interaction [41] mainly relied on wearable tracking systems. Hand gestures could be captured through movement sensors, including *data gloves* that precisely track movements of user's hand and fingers. Yanbin et al. [42] proposed a virtual simulation to train nurses and midwifes in accomplishing operations. The system used data gloves to track hands movement of trainees and created 3D reconstructions to assess difficult childbirth situations.

Computer vision (CV) techniques play a fundamental role in enabling natural interaction through hands tracking and body gesture recognition [43]. CV systems allow to capture user interaction in a completely non-intrusive and passive manner and can therefore represent an effective and low-cost technology in medical application and simulations in general [44]. Furthermore, CV systems can reduce required device capabilities and cost. Advanced pattern recognition pipelines in fact allow to sense user actions (e.g., the hand gestures used in our prototypes) through commercially available low-cost cameras. At the same time, cameras used for hand gesture recognition can be used for other interface functionalities. Hand gesture-based application has found use in different contexts in the medical field. In [45], authors introduced a CV-based application to let surgeons interact with computing devices through hand gestures. This allowed medical image visualization in the operating room without the need of touching any input device.

In the last decade, the introduction of low-cost depth cameras such as the Microsoft Kinect™ has paved the road for the development of increasingly more interactive simulator. Depth cameras allow a more robust tracking of the scene and of the user, making possible to implement novel ways of user interaction with computer interfaces. Kinect-enabled systems have been commonly used in medical rehabilitation. Lange et al. [46], for example, have developed a Kinect-based game "JewelMine" that consists of a set of balance training exercises to stimulate the players to reach out of their base of support. This kind of software takes advantage of the situation realism and the naturalness allowed by the Kinect sensor in gestures tracking. This is relevant especially to encourage physical exercise but it is an approach not quite common in medical operators training systems. LISSA [47] is a Kinect-based system developed to train specific skills in Cardiopulmonary Resuscitation (CPR). This system is one of the first medical training software exploiting motion tracking but compared to BLSD-S, our prototype presented in Sect. 4.2.2, LISSA is more skill-oriented rather than procedure-oriented.

In this book, we show how computer vision can be exploited in NI-enabled VR systems augmenting the capabilities of state-of-the-art devices such as the Microsoft Kinect™ on which our prototypes rely on. Hand gesture recognition is used to simplify interactions in the BLSD-S prototype (see Sect. 4.2.2). Automatic user's recognition obtained with CV algorithms is exploited to associate users to simulation roles (e.g., simulation that differentiates roles such as surgeon or nurse) and to re-identify the user in order to keep track of his/her performances in our Surgical Safety Checklist simulator (see Sect. 4.3). Dedicated hand-tracking cameras such as Leap Motion also represent a solid and low-cost solution to create gesture-based simulators using embedded tracking software. An example of this technology can be found in [48], where a gesture-based cataract surgery simulation is presented. We also exploit the Leap Motion in an advanced version of our BLSD-S (II) prototype, presented in Sect. 4.2.9.

2.3.2 Virtual Reality: New Perspectives

Virtual reality (VR) applications in the medical field have seen a growing interests. Although VR technology has been around for more than a decade, latest improvement in commercial hardware has greatly increased the possibility of new applications in critical fields. Nowadays, novel head-mounted displays (HMDs), such as the Oculus Rift or the Samsung Gear, offer very high-resolution graphics, low-latency performance, and accurate head tracking systems, allowing user to have a really realistic and immersive experience. More than two decades ago, Satava [41] proposed a pioneer application of virtual reality in medical simulation for anatomy lesson and surgical procedure simulation. The application adopted an early version of an HMD and sensorized gloves as a hand tracker input device. In his system evaluation, Satava highlighted two of the most critical limitations of VR technologies at that time: (1) The 3D computer graphics reduced the likelihood of the simulation caused by the low quality of the rendering, and (2) the limited resolution of the HMD decreased the quality of the visualization. Almost ten years after the first prototype of Satava, a randomized double-blind study was conducted [49] to assess the effect of VR training system in operating room performance. In the study, it was shown that students that were trained using a VR simulator significantly improved the performance during a laparoscopic cholecystectomy procedure. The improvement was attributable to the likelihood of the simulation and to the fact that this type of simulation and the isolation induced increases the level of concentration of the user.

As argued in a recent survey [50], many virtual reality simulators exploiting these new devices have been standardized and validated, showing clear positive outcomes in the medical training. As a quite valuable example, Vankipuram et al. [51] proposed a VR-based training simulator for advanced cardiac life support. The chosen scenario is a pretty common one in medical simulation, since it allows to simulate skills such as situational awareness and team cooperation in a critical situation and has some similarities to our BLSD-S prototype, presented in Sect. 4.2.2.

In concluding this chapter, it is important to point out that VR systems exploiting NI technologies can help trainees to develop certain skills in a safe and realistic environment, using natural gestures, and allow multiple repetitions of the simulation with no additional costs. However, it has to be clear that not every procedure equally

Table 2.1 Solutions adopt+ed by the different medical simulation systems

	Visualization			Interaction		
	3D Graphics	Immersive env	Virtual Reality	Mouse and Keyboard	Haptic device	Gesture-based
Cybermed [7]	✓			✓	✓	
SOFA [8]	✓			✓		
ViMet [9]	✓			✓	✓	
GiPSi [12]	✓	✓			✓	
Honey et al. [15]	✓	✓		✓		
Cowan et al. [16]	✓	✓		✓		
Spring [10]	✓	✓		✓		
JDoc [17]	✓	✓		✓		
Microsim [11]				✓		
Yanbin et al. [42]	✓					✓
Buttussi et al. [18]	✓	✓		✓		
LISSA [47]	✓					✓
Jayakumar et al. [48]	✓			✓		✓
Satava [41]	✓		✓			✓
Vankipuram et al. [51]	✓	✓	✓		✓	

benefits from such technologies. In fact, while the quality of the computer graphic is constantly improving and has reached a broadly accepted level of realism, interaction is still an issue with many simulators. In some scenarios, such as a surgical operation, simulator needs to provide a tactile feedback to the trainees in order for them to have real feeling of the tissue. In other cases, such as eye surgery or an intubation procedure, users need to perform actions that require a very high accuracy in activities understanding. In these scenarios, haptic devices are generally preferred to purely virtual methods which, anyway, are the main subject of this book and are discussed in Chap. 4.

In the next chapter, are presented in detail the computer vision methods for re-identification and the gesture recognition modules that have been used in our prototypes to improve interaction design and systems usability.

References

1. Harris SB (1992) The society for the recovery of persons apparently dead. Skept 24–31
2. Cooper J, Taqueti VR (2004) A brief history of the development of mannequin simulators for clinical education and training. Qual Saf Health Care
3. Gaba DM (2004) The future vision of simulation in health care, Qual Saf Health Care

4. Bradley P (2006) The history of simulation in medical education and possible future directions. Med Educ
5. McIntosh C, Macario A, Flanagan B, Gaba D (2006) Simulation: what does it really cost?. Simul Healthc J Soc Simul Healthc
6. Dale E (1969) Audio-visual methods in teaching. Holt(Rinehart and Winston), NY, USA
7. Sales BRA, Machado LS, Moraes RM (2011) Interactive collaboration for virtual reality systems related to medical education and training. CRC Press, Technology and Medical Sciences, pp 157–162
8. Allard J, Cotin S, Faure F, Bensoussan PJ, Poyer F, Duriez C et al (2007) SOFA—an open source framework for medical simulation. Med Meets Virtual Real 15:1–6
9. Oliveira ACMTG, Botega LC, Pavarini L, Rossatto DJ, Nunes FLS, Bezerra A (2006) Virtual reality framework for medical training: implementation of a deformation class using Java. In: Proceedings of the SIGGRAPH international conference on virtual-reality continuum and its applications in industry (SIGGRAPH 2006). T.F.H. (Publications), Hong Kong, pp. 347–351
10. Montgomery K, Bruyns C, Brown J, Sorkin S, Mazzella F, Thonier G, Tellier A, Lerman B, Menon A (2002) Spring: a general framework for collaborative, real-time surgical simulation. Med Meets Virtual Real (MMVR) 23–26
11. MicroSim L (2012). http://www.laerdal.com/it/docid/5899175/MicroSim
12. Goktekin T, Cavusoglu MC, Tendick F, Sastry S (2004) GiPSi: an open source open architecture software development framework for surgical simulation. In: Proceedings of the international symposium on medical simulation. Cambridge
13. Kononowicz AA et al (2012) Effects of introducing a voluntary virtual patient module to a basic life support with an automated external defibrillator course: a randomised trial. BMC Med Educ 12(1):41
14. Kelle S, Klemke R, Specht M (2013) Effects of game design patterns on basic life support training content. Int Forum Educ Technol Soc (IFETS)
15. Honey MLL, Diener S, Connor K, Veltman M, Bodily D (2009) Teaching in virtual space: second life simulation for haemorrhage management. In: Ascilite Conference. Aukland
16. Cowan B, Shelley M, Sabri H, Kapralos B, Hogue A, Hogan M, Jenkin M, Goldsworthy G, Rose L, Dubrowski A (2008) Interprofessional care simulator for critical care education. In: Proceedings of the 2008 conference on future play: research, play, share (Future Play-08). ACM, New York, NY, USA, pp 260–261
17. Sliney A, Murphy D (2008) Jdoc: a serious game for medical learning. In: International conference on advances in computer-human interaction
18. Buttussi F, Pellis T, Cabas VA, Pausler D, Carchietti E, Chittaro L (2013) Evaluation of a 3D serious game for advanced life support retraining. Int J Med Inf. Elsevier
19. Abt CC (1987) Serious games. University press of America
20. Hansen MM (2008) Versatile, immersive, creative and dynamic virtual 3-D healthcare learning environments: a review of the literature. J Med Internet Res 10(3)
21. Schreuder HW, Oei G, Maas M, Borleffs JC, Schijven MP (2011) Implementation of simulation in surgical practice: minimally invasive surgery has taken the lead: the Dutch experience. Med Teach 33(2):105–115
22. Cook DA, Hatala R, Brydges R, Zendejas B, Szostek JH, Wang AT, Erwin PJ, Hamstra SJ (2011) Technology-enhanced simulation for health professions education: a systematic review and meta-analysis. JAMA 306(9):978–988
23. Cowan B, Sabri H, Kapralos B, Moussa F, Cristancho S, Dubrowski A (2011) A serious game for off-pump coronary artery bypass surgery procedure training. In: MMVR, pp 147–149
24. Cowan B, Sabri H, Kapralos B, Porte M, Backstein D, Cristancho S, Dubrowski A (2010) A serious game for total knee arthroplasty procedure, education and training. J Cyber Ther Rehabil 3(3):285–98
25. Bowyer MW, Streete KA, Muniz GM, Liu AV (2008) Immersive virtual environments for medical training. In: Seminars in colon and rectal surgery 2008 Jun 30 (vol 19, no 2). WB Saunders, Philadelphia, PA, USA, pp 90–97

26. Andreatta PB, Maslowski E, Petty S, Shim W, Marsh M, Hall T, Stern S, Frankel J (2010) Virtual reality triage training provides a viable solution for disaster preparedness. Acad Emerg Med 17(8):870–876
27. Kurenov SN, Cance WW, Noel B, Mozingo DW (2008) Game-based mass casualty burn training. Stud Health Tech Inf 142:142–4
28. Parvati DE, Heinrichs WL, Patricia Y (2011) CliniSpace: a multiperson 3D online immersive training environment accessible through a browser. Med Meets Virtual Real 18 NextMed 163:173
29. Taekman JM, Shelley K (2010) Virtual environments in healthcare: immersion, disruption, and flow. Int Anesthesiol Clin 48(3):101–121
30. Youngblood P, Harter PM, Srivastava S, Moffett S, Heinrichs WL, Dev P (2008) Design, development, and evaluation of an online virtual emergency department for training trauma teams. Simul Healthc 3(3):146–53
31. Heinrichs WL, Youngblood P, Harter PM, Dev P (2008) Simulation for team training and assessment: case studies of online training with virtual worlds. World J Surg 32(2):161–170
32. Wiederhold BK, Wiederhold MD (2008) Virtual reality for posttraumatic stress disorder and stress inoculation training. J CyberTher Rehabil 1(1):23–35
33. Alverson DC, Saiki SM Jr, Caudell TP, Summers K, Panaiotis, Sherstyuk A, Nickles D, Holten J, Goldsmith T, Stevens S, Kihmm K, Mennin S, Kalishman S, Mines J, Serna L, Mitchell S, Lindberg M, Jacobs J, Nakatsu C, Lozanoff S, Wax DS, Saland L, Norenberg J, Shuster G, Keep M, Baker R, Buchanan HS, Stewart R, Bowyer M, Liu A, Muniz G, Coulter R, Maris C, Wilks D (2005) Distributed immersive virtual reality simulation development for medical education, J Int Assoc Med Sci Educ 15–1
34. Kaufman M (2006) Team training of medical first responders for CBRNE events using multiplayer game technology. In: Proceedings of medicine meets virtual reality
35. Duffy TM, Jonassen DH (1992) Constructivism and the technology of instruction, Constructivism: new implications for instructional technology. A conversation. pp 1–6
36. Hogle JG. Considering games as cognitive tools: in search of effective
37. Luo X et al (2005) Integration of augmented reality and assistive devices for post-stroke hand opening rehabilitation. In: Proceedings of IEEE engineering in medicine and biology 27th annual conference. pp 6855–6858
38. Gunn C, Hutchins M, Stevenson D, Adcock M, Youngblood P (2005) Using collaborative haptics in remote surgical training. In: Eurohaptics conference and symposium on haptic interfaces for virtual environment and teleoperator systems (WHC2005). Italy
39. Burke JW, McNeill MDJ, Charles DK, Morrow PJ, Crosbie JH, McDonough SM (2010) Augmented reality games for upper-limb stroke rehabilitation. In: 2010 second international conference on games and virtual worlds for serious applications (VS-GAMES). IEEE, pp 75–78
40. Sparks D, Chase D, Coughlin L (2009) Wii have a problem: a review of self- reported Wii related injuries. Inform Prim Care 17(1):55–57
41. Satava RM (1993) Virtual reality surgical simulator. Surg Endosc 7(3):203–205
42. Yanbin P, Hanwu H, Jinfang L, Dali Z (2007) Data-glove based interactive training system for virtual delivery operation. In: Second workshop on digital media and its application in museum and heritages. IEEE, pp 383–388
43. Wachs JP, Klsch M, Stern H, Edan Y (2011) Vision-based hand-gesture applications. Commun ACM 54(2):60–71
44. Rautaray SS, Agrawal A (2015) Vision based hand gesture recognition for human computer interaction: a survey. Artif Intell Rev 43(1):1–54
45. Graetzel C, Fong T, Grange S, Baur C (2004) A non-contact mouse for surgeon-computer interaction. Technol Health Care 12(3):245–257
46. Lange B, Koenig S, McConnell E, Chang C, Juang R, Suma E, Bolas M, Rizzo A (2012) Interactive game-based rehabilitation using the Microsoft kinect. Virtual reality short papers and posters (VRW), IEEE
47. Wattanasoontorn V, Magdics M, Boada I, Sbert M (2013). A kinect-based system for cardiopulmonary resuscitation simulation: a pilot study. In: Serious games development and applications. Springer Berlin Heidelberg, pp 51–63

48. Jayakumar A, Mathew B, Uma N, Nedungadi P (2015) Interactive gesture based cataract surgery simulation. In: 2015 Fifth international conference on advances in computing and communications (ICACC). IEEE, pp 350–353

49. Seymour NE, Gallagher AG, Roman SA, O'brien, MK, Bansal VK, Andersen DK, Satava RM (2002) Virtual reality training improves operating room performance: results of a randomized, double-blinded study. Ann Surg 236(4):458

50. Ruthenbeck Greg S, Reynolds Karen J (2015) Virtual reality for medical training: the state-of-the-art. J Simul 9(1):16–26

51. Vankipuram A, Khanal P, Ashby A, Vankipuram M, Gupta A, DrummGurnee D, Josey K, Smith M (2014) Design and development of a virtual reality simulator for advanced cardiac life support training. IEEE J Biomed Health Inform 18(4):1478–1484

Chapter 3
Computer Vision for Natural Interfaces

Abstract Depth cameras simplify many tasks in computer vision, such as background modeling, 3D reconstruction, articulated object tracking, and gesture analysis. These sensors provide a great tool for real-time analysis of human behavior. In this chapter, we cover two important issues that can be solved using computer vision for natural interaction. First, we show how we can address the issue of coarse hand pose recognition at a distance, allowing a user to perform common gestures such as picking, dragging, and clicking without the aid of any remote. Second, we deal with the challenging task of long-term re-identification. In the typical approach, person re-identification is performed using appearance, thus invalidating any application in which a person may change dress across subsequent acquisitions. For example, this is a relevant scenario for home patient monitoring. Unfortunately, face and skeleton quality is not always enough to grant a correct recognition from depth data. Both features are affected by the pose of the subject and the distance from the camera. We propose a model to incorporate a robust skeleton representation with a highly discriminative face feature, weighting samples by their quality (Part of this chapter previously appeared in Bagdanov et al. (Real-time hand status recognition from RGB-D imagery, pp. 2456–2012 [1]) and in Bondi et al. (Long termperson re-identification 488 from depth cameras using facial and skeleton data, 2016 [2]) with permission of Springer.).

Keywords Computer vision · RGB-D imaging · Hand recognition · Face recognition

3.1 Introduction

Advances in 3D scanning technologies make it possible to capture geometric and visual data of an observed scene and its dynamics across time. The availability of registered depth and RGB frames across time boosts the potential of automatic analysis modules that can now easily detect and track people and their body parts as they move in the scene.

However, the technologies employed in current 3D dynamic scanning devices limit their field of view at a distance of a few meters, with the quality of the sensed data

© The Author(s) 2017
A. Del Bimbo et al., *Natural Interaction in Medical Training*, SpringerBriefs in Human-Computer Interaction,
https://doi.org/10.1007/978-3-319-61036-8_3

degrading already at 2 m distance. As a consequence, the tracking libraries released with such devices can track the target just if it is visible and sufficiently close to the sensor. Moreover, finer joints, such as fingers, can be hardly tracked at distances farther than 1 m. This issue makes it challenging to deploy computer vision systems, employing RGB-D sensors, in natural interactive environments. However, existing RGB-D processing SDKs can be augmented with pattern recognition modules adding these important functionalities.

Despite the ability to track a human body in real time, the implementation of generic user interfaces remains an open problem. An accurate skeletal configuration enables game and application designers to improve the quality of interaction. Users can control a virtual self directly, and basic activities can be recognized just by comparing the sequence of body configurations with existing templates. Nevertheless, some classic user interaction paradigms are lacking. Classical gesture analysis approaches go a long way toward addressing these needs [3], but access to real-time depth imagery opens new horizons.

Applications that require pointing, clicking, drag-and-drop, and all of the gestures that stem from this basic vocabulary are not generally supported by body-driven platforms. The main issue is the difficulty of adding a state to the coordinates of the body without constraining the user position in space. The usual work-around is based on[1] persistence: A user must keep her arm still for a not-so-short span of time while pointing at an object which she wants to interact with. This kind of interaction is usually limited to sections of an application where the user spends less than 5% of her time—like a setup menu or the start screen of an application. We propose to overcome this limitation and improve interface reactivity by employing a vision module able to recognize simple hand poses in order to add a state to the virtual pointer represented by the user hand.

Recognition of hand poses and gestures with depth imagery has been addressed in the past. Oikonomidis et al. developed a tracker for an articulated hand model using a particle swarm optimization [5]. Their technique is computationally extremely expensive and requires GPU acceleration. Moreover, their benchmark is conducted on synthetic data, and as far we can determine there are no results (even qualitative) that show the system tracking hands at a distance larger than 1 m. Suryanarayan et al. [6] proposed a compressed 3D shape descriptor computed on depth images of hands. They state that the interaction distance is set to 1.5 m. Finally, Ren et al. [7] defined a finger Earth Mover's Distance that allows partial matching of segmented hand shapes. Their system works at close distances, but requires the user to wear a black wrist band in order to correctly segment the hand.

Another compelling feature is the possibility to recognize users continuously even when they exit the scene or in case they use the system at different times, possibly with different outfits. If the moving target becomes too far from the sensor or it is no more in its field of view, tracking is not possible. The ultimate result is that, in the case a target

---

[1] Part of this chapter previously appeared in [4] ©2014 Association for Computing Machinery, Inc. Reprinted by permission.

observed in the past enters again the field of view of the camera, it is considered as a new one, loosing any relation between the two intervals of observation.

Consider a multi-user complex simulation which requires different users to take part at different times. For medical training, it is not uncommon that each team member has a specific role, paramedic, medical doctor as it will be shown in our case studies in Chap. 4. A system designed to train and monitor the correct behavior and performance of multi-role teams has the need to re-identify possibly lost users during a conceited activity.

Another interesting scenario related to the medical field is the monitoring of a patient in a domestic environment. This is desirable in the case of elderly people or persons following a rehabilitation program at home. Suppose we want to monitor the long-term behavior of the patient using one or multiple 3D sensors (like Kinect camera), each of them with a field of view constrained to a room or part of it. The ultimate goal of such a system could be the extraction of indices of position, movement, action, and behavior of the patient along days or weeks. This requires the correct identification of the monitored subject through subsequent temporal intervals, in which he/she is visible in the field of view of the cameras. Change in the appearance of the target subject as well as the presence of multiple persons should be also accounted for.

The task of person re-identification consists in recognizing an individual in different locations over a set of non-overlapping camera views. Re-identification from depth images is facilitated by the joint face and body measurement. However, these measurements are far from accurate when using low-cost sensors, such as Kinect. First, face imagery allows a face reconstruction via super-resolution only if a sufficient amount of views with enough resolution is available. On the other hand, skeleton is not always correctly estimated. Pose and distance may affect the accuracy of joints location estimation. Back and profile poses cause imprecise estimations. Moreover, when a subject is too close to the camera, many joints are occluded causing an almost total failure in the body feature computation. Figure 3.1 shows critical situations for both face and skeleton acquisitions.

In Sect. 3.3, we will describe a model which deals with these issues and allows us to perform re-identification accurately even if one of the two biometric cues is missing or inaccurately computed.

Re-identification approaches have been developed first using 2D videos. Most of these 2D solutions rely on appearance-based only techniques, which assume that individuals do not change their clothing during the observation period [8, 9]. This hypothesis constrains such re-identification methods to be applied under a limited temporal range.

Recently, the use of biometric features has been considered as viable solution to overcome such limitations. In particular, there is an increasing interest in performing person re-identification using 3D data. This idea has been first exploited using 3D soft-biometric features. For example, Velardo and Dugelay [10] used anthropometric data obtained in a strongly supervised scenario, where a complete cooperation of the user is required to take manual measures of the body. However, in order to extend the applicability of re-identification systems to more practical scenarios, they should deal with subjects that do not explicitly cooperate with the system. This has been made

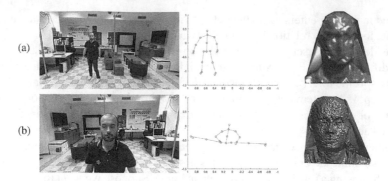

Fig. 3.1 Examples of skeleton and face mesh (Florence 3D Re-Id dataset): **a** For a far person (3 m), the skeleton is estimated correctly, while the face mesh has very low quality; **b** for a close person (0.8 m), leg joints are wrongly estimated, while the face mesh is noisy, but has high resolution

possible thanks to the introduction of low-cost 3D cameras capable of acquiring metric data of moving subjects in a dynamic way.

Several recent works exploited the opportunities given by such devices and performed person re-identification using soft-biometric cues. In [11], Barbosa et al. presented a set of 3D soft-biometric cues that are gathered using RGB-D technology and being insensitive to appearance variations can be used for person re-identification. These include skeleton-based features (i.e., distances between joints of the skeleton, ratio between joint distances, and distances between joints and floor) and surface-based features (i.e., geodesic distances between joints computed on the reconstructed surface of the subject's 3D model). The joint use of these characteristics provides encouraging performances on a benchmark of 79 people that have been captured in different days and with different clothing. This promotes a novel research direction for the re-identification community, supported also by the fact that a new brand of affordable RGB-D cameras has recently invaded the worldwide market.

Pala et al. [12] investigated whether the re-identification accuracy of clothing appearance descriptors can be improved by fusing them with anthropometric measures extracted from depth data, using RGB-D sensors, in unconstrained settings. Satta et al. [13] investigate the deployment of real-world re-identification systems, by developing and testing a working prototype. The focus of this work is on two practical issues: computational complexity, and reliability of segmentation and tracking. The former is addressed by using a recently proposed fast re-identification method, the latter by using Kinect cameras.

Baltieri et al. [14] proposed a re-identification framework, which exploits non-articulated 3D body models to spatially map appearance descriptors (color and gradient histograms) into the vertices of a regularly sampled 3D body surface. The matching and the shot integration steps are directly handled in the 3D body model, reducing the effects of occlusions, partial views, or pose changes, which normally afflict 2D descriptors. A fast and effective model-to-image alignment is also proposed. It allows operation on common surveillance cameras or image collections. A comprehensive experimental evaluation is presented using the benchmark suite 3DPeS.

In [15], Munaro et al. proposed a method for creating 3D models of persons freely moving in front of a consumer depth sensor and show how they can be used for long-term person re-identification. To overcome the problem of the different poses a person can assume, the information provided by skeletal tracking algorithms is exploited for warping every point cloud frame to a standard pose in real time. Then, the warped point clouds are merged together to compose the model. Re-identification is performed by matching body shapes in terms of whole point clouds warped to a standard pose with the described method. The technique is compared with a classification method based on a descriptor of skeleton features and with a mixed approach which exploits both skeleton and shape features. Experiments are reported on two datasets acquired for RGB-D re-identification which use different skeletal tracking algorithms and which are made publicly available to foster research in this new research branch.

In this chapter, we show two effective solutions, based on computer vision, to enable standard RGB-D processing pipeline to perform hand gestures at a distance and to correctly recognize users fusing face and skeletal features (Fig. 3.2).

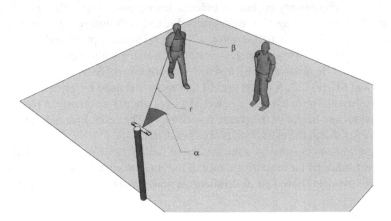

Fig. 3.2 *Reference system.* The subject position is accounted through the distance r measured along the ray connecting the camera to the subject, and the angles α and β formed by the ray and the viewing direction of, respectively, the camera and the subject

3.2 Hand Pose Recognition

In this section, we detail how to represent images robustly in sequences captured from RGB-D devices, and how we can, in real-time, obtain a simple status of the hand enabling a rich vocabulary of interaction gesture even at extreme distances.

The first step in our hand status recognizer is the segmentation of hand regions from the background. Given the real-world center of mass coordinates of a hand $\overline{h}$, we threshold the user map M_u with a value of $D_h + 10\,\mathrm{cm}$ where D_h is the depth at the center of mass of the hand. In this way, we obtain the hand map M_h. Finally, the binary image M_h is projected in the RGB coordinate system to extract only the pixels of the user hand. M_u is obtained by applying background subtraction to the depth sequence, while $\overline{h}$ can be obtained by averaging the pixel coordinates of the hand body part detected using [16] or performing a double thresholding on the depth image and extracting only pixels $p_h \in \left[\overline{D_u} + \delta, \max(D_u)\right]$, where D_u are the depth pixels of a user and $\overline{D_u}$ is her center of mass. We found $\delta = 15\,\mathrm{cm}$ to be a reasonable setting for all users.

3.2.1 Hand Representation

We conducted a preliminary evaluation of local descriptors and spatial configurations on a small dataset consisting of three subjects. We tested the following spatial configurations: a single whole-patch descriptor, a 2×2 grid of descriptors, and a 2×2 grid plus a central location (five subpatches in total). For individual descriptors, we tested SIFT [17], global Hu moments [18], and the two variations of SURF descriptors [19]: SURF-64 and SURF-128. A dense grid of features is obtained by extracting patches with 50% overlap. The patch size is selected as $\frac{2}{3}r$, where $r = min(w, h)$ and w and h are the width and height of the patch, respectively. The central patch has the same size. Figure 3.3 shows the extraction process in detail.

In our preliminary evaluation, summarized in Table 3.1, SIFT and both SURF versions outperformed by far the performance of the Hu moments. This is not surprising, since the Hu moments have less discriminative power and are mainly shape descrip-

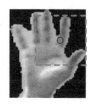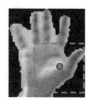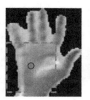

Fig. 3.3 Feature extraction procedure

Table 3.1 Features and spatial layout

Feat.	Conf.		
	1 (%)	2 × 2	2 × 2 + 1
Hu	56.00	–	–
SIFT	82.97	–	–
SURF-64	83.63	86.12%	86.96%
SURF-128	86.92	86.79%	**87.81%**

tors. Shape can be discriminative only at high resolutions (distance < 1.5 m), while at farther distances shape becomes more ambiguous.

SURF-64 performed slightly worse than SURF-128, but both SURF variations had an edge on SIFT. SIFT descriptors are probably too discriminative, and their more detailed representation of the pattern generated more noise. The single patch representation was outperformed by grid configurations, and in particular the $2 \times 2 + 1$ configuration was the one that gave the best results. The final hand representation is computed as the concatenation of the five SURF-128 descriptors for a total of 640 dimensions.

3.2.2 Hand Status Recognition

For hand status recognition, we train a support vector machine (SVM) with a nonlinear RBF kernel of the form $k(x, y) = \exp(-\gamma ||x - y||^2)$. The C regularization parameter and the γ kernel parameter are determined through a fivefold cross-validation procedure on the training set. The distance of a test sample x to the SVM decision margin is:

$$f(x) = \sum_i \alpha_i y_i k(x_i, x),$$ (3.1)

where x_i are the support vectors (SVs), y_i are their labels (+1 open, −1 closed), and α_i are the SV weights.

In practice, we noticed that the SVM output $f(x)$ is quite noisy (see Fig. 3.9 for an example). Consequently, we model the SVM classification function as a noisy measurement process of the true hand state at time k: $f_k(x) = f_{k-1}(x) + \sigma$, where σ is a zero-mean, Gaussian noise term. The SVM output at time k is used to update a Kalman filter that estimates $f_k(x)$. The sign of $f_k(x)$ is then the smoothed predictor of the current hand status. As shown in Fig. 3.4, the classifier output smoothly follows the hand status.

Thus, we suppose that a model trained on some reasonably descriptive data will be affected by an error with a Gaussian distribution $\mathcal{N}(0, \sigma)$.

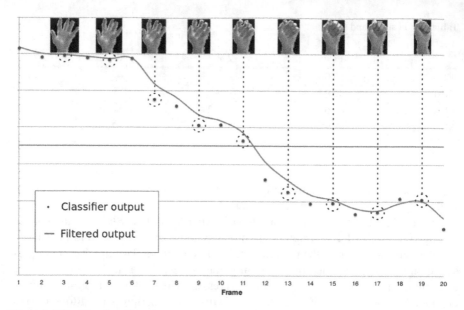

Fig. 3.4 Filtered and unfiltered output

The hand state is the state of a dynamical system with the following equation: $x(k + 1) = x(k) + v$, where v is a Gaussian noise. This means that the hand state tends not to change too abruptly. This assumption is reasonable if the system is able to obtain high frame rate imagery (15 Hz).

3.3 Long-Term Re-identification

In this section, we deal with the challenging problem of long-term re-identification. We exploit 3D face models and 3D skeletal features. Face meshes captured from RGB-D devices are often noisy and require super-resolution in order to obtain a reliable recognition result. Nonetheless, at farther distances faces become unreliable and skeletal feature comes into play. We exploit a cumulated observed model to aggregate features from subsequent frames for faces and skeletons. The fusion of both features improves recognition results, making it feasible to recognize users both at close and far distances.

3.3.1 Cumulated Observed Model

The system setup features a Kinect v2.0 camera mounted on a vertical pole at approximately 2 m from the ground and oriented so as to observe people entering and moving in a room (see the *reference system* in Fig. 3.2). Using the Kinect SDK, the camera outputs RGB and depth frames as well as the 3D coordinates and orientation of the skeleton joints, for up to six persons. These data are processed to compute the position and orientation of a generic subject within the field of view of the camera in terms of *radial distance r*, the *azimuthal angle* α, and the *yaw angle* β (see Fig. 3.2). Pitch and roll angles, although provided by the SDK, are presently not considered.

Values of (r, α, β) are discretized so as to represent the position and orientation of a generic subject with respect to the camera by using the triple (i, j, k) to index one among N_c possible configurations. Given the observation (r, α, β) representing the position and orientation of a generic subject with respect to the camera, quantized observed configuration indexes (i_o, j_o, k_o) are computed as:

$$
\begin{cases}
i_o = \arg\min_i |r_i - r| \,, & i = \{1, \ldots, N_r\} \\
j_o = \arg\min_j |\alpha_j - \alpha| \,, & j = \{1, \ldots, N_\alpha\} \\
k_o = \arg\min_k |\beta_k - \beta| \,, & k = \{1, \ldots, N_\beta\} \,.
\end{cases}
\tag{3.2}
$$

For a generic observation, a confidence measure is estimated to express the presence of out of focus artifacts in the RGB data caused by subject motion or inadequate lighting. In this way, a new observation with quantized configuration indexes (i_o, j_o, k_o) replaces the previous observation with the same quantized configuration indexes only if the confidence of the new observation is greater than the confidence of the previous one. Figure 3.5 shows an example of the observations retained after tracking a subject who wandered in front of the camera for some time.

In addition to this multi-view representation of the face, the Cumulative Observation Model (COM) retains a representation of the skeleton of the observed person. This is achieved by computing an exponential moving average measure of the distance between some pairs of body joints.

By adopting an exponential weighted moving average measure of the body parts, the accuracy of the skeleton-based representation of the observed person increases with the duration of the observation. This enables the use of these data to complement facial data and increase the accuracy of re-identification.

We weigh each skeletal descriptor according to our reliability function:

$$
r(s) = \frac{|\mathcal{J}_T|}{|\mathcal{J}|} + \frac{1}{2} \cdot (1 - \mathbf{z} \cdot \mathbf{v}) + \frac{\|\text{head} - \text{head}_{gp}\|}{H_{geo}} \,.
\tag{3.3}
$$

The reliability function $r(s)$ has three terms:

- $\frac{|\mathcal{J}_T|}{|\mathcal{J}|}$ takes into account the reliability of the joint tracking by computing the ratio of tracked joints $j \in \mathcal{J}_T$ with respect to the whole joint set $\mathcal{J}$.

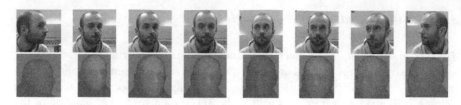

Fig. 3.5 Example of representative views of a subject retained by the Cumulative Observation Model (Florence 3D Re-Id dataset)

- $\frac{1}{2} \cdot (1 - \mathbf{z} \cdot \mathbf{v})$ evaluates the body pose, where $\mathbf{z}$ is the vector indicating the z-axis in the camera reference and $\mathbf{v}$ is the vector perpendicular to the plane estimated from torso joints.
- $\frac{||\text{head}-\text{head}_{gp}||}{H_{geo}}$ evaluates how *erected* a subject pose is. H_{geo} is the geodesic height, defined as:

$$H_{geo} = ||\text{head} - \text{neck}|| + ||\text{spine-mid} - \text{spine-base}|| +$$
$$\frac{1}{2}(||\text{left-hip} - \text{left-knee}|| + ||\text{lknee} - \text{lankle}|| +$$
$$||\text{rhip} - \text{rknee}|| + ||\text{rknee} - \text{rankle}||) \,,$$

where head_{gp} is the projection of the head onto the ground plane. Note that in computing H_{geo}, we average on the leg lengths for improved accuracy. Considering a skeleton descriptor at frame t, s_t, we compute the cumulated observation for a sequence of skeletons $\mathscr{S}$ as:

$$s^* = \sum_{s_t \in \mathscr{S}} d_\alpha(t) \cdot r(s_t) \cdot s \,, \tag{3.4}$$

where $d_\alpha(t) = \exp\left(\frac{t}{\tau}\right)$ is an exponential decay term that weights decreasingly the relevance of descriptors s_t.

3.3.2 Super-Resolved Face Model

Observations retained from different viewpoints by the COM are used to build a 3D model of the face of the subject using a 3D super-resolution approach, developing on the model proposed in [20].

Each range image retained by the COM is converted into a point cloud, and information about the acquisition radius, azimuth, and yaw angles is used to roughly align the different point clouds to a common (X, Y, Z) reference system. The Iterative Closest Point (ICP) algorithm [21] is then used for fine registration of the point clouds with respect to each other. For each point, its (X, Y, Z) coordinates as well as the direction of the scanner line of sight for that point are retained. This latter is used to account for the anisotropic error distribution in the approximation of the face surface. Once all the point clouds are registered and aligned to a common reference system, estimation of the face surface is operated by fitting a mean face model to the data (points of the clouds). This is performed in two steps: mean face model alignment and mean face model warping. The ICP algorithm is used for alignment, whereas warping is accomplished by updating the coordinates of each vertex of the mean face model based on the spatial distribution of the closest points of the cloud. The deformable face model proposed in [22] is used as mean face model.

Formally, considering one generic vertex $\mathbf{v} = (v_x, v_y, v_z)$ of the mean face model, the subset of the point cloud (PC) composed of points within a range Δ from the vertex is considered:

$$\mathscr{S}(\mathbf{v}) = \{\mathbf{x} \in PC \mid \|\mathbf{v} - \mathbf{x}\| < \Delta\} .$$ (3.5)

Each point $\mathbf{x}_i \in \mathscr{S}(\mathbf{v})$ is assigned a weight w_i accounting for its distance to $\mathbf{v}$. Eventually, the coordinates of $\mathbf{v}$ are updated through the following expression:

$$\mathbf{v} = \frac{\sum w_i \mathbf{x}_i}{\sum w_i} .$$ (3.6)

Figure 3.6 shows two sample facial point clouds retained by the COM, the cumulated facial point cloud obtained by registering all the retained point clouds, the mean face model before and after the warping process.

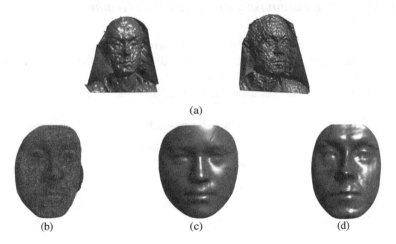

Fig. 3.6 Construction of the face model using observations from multiple viewpoints. Two sample facial point clouds retained by the COM (**a**), the cumulated facial point cloud obtained by registering all the retained point clouds (**b**), the mean face model before (**c**) and after (**d**) the warping process

3.3.3   Re-identification Based on Face Geometry

Re-identification based on face geometry operates by reconstructing a 3D face model of each observed person and matching this probe against a gallery set composed of reconstructed 3D face models of previously observed persons. In the case a match is found the person is re-identified. Description and matching of gallery and probe models is obtained according to the approach proposed in [23] that is based on the extraction and comparison of local features of the face. First, SIFT keypoints of the face are detected and a subset of them is retained by applying a hierarchical clustering. In this way, a cluster of keypoints with similar position and SIFT descriptors is substituted by a 'representative keypoint,' thus reducing the overall number of keypoints. Then, the relational information between representative keypoints is captured by measuring how the face geometry changes along the surface path connecting pairs of keypoints. By sectioning the face through a plane passing from the two keypoints and orthogonal to the surface, a *facial curve* is extracted. Face similarity is evaluated by finding correspondences between keypoints of probe and gallery scans, and matching the facial curves across the inlier pairs of matching keypoints. The approach revealed good performance across different datasets and also in the case of partial face matching. This provides the 3D face recognition approach with the required robustness to manage our scenario.

3.3.4   Re-identification Based on Body Part Geometry

Considering the fact that arms and legs are often wrongly located by Kinect, we only rely on features computed from the torso. Indeed, knees and hands have the lowest recognition rate [24]. We use neck, spine, shoulders, and hips, and specifically we compute the following features using Euclidean distances:

$$s^{ns} = ||\text{neck} - \text{spine-mid}||,$$
$$s^{mb} = ||\text{spine-mid} - \text{spine-base}||$$
$$s^{nls} = ||\text{neck} - \text{lshould}||$$
$$s^{nrs} = ||\text{neck} - \text{lshould}||$$
$$s^{lhb} = ||\text{lhip} - \text{spine-base}||$$
$$s^{rhb} = ||\text{rhip} - \text{spine-base}||$$
$$s^{mls} = ||\text{spine-mid} - \text{lshould}||$$
$$s^{mrs} = ||\text{spine-mid} - \text{rshould}|| .$$

For a skeleton at time t, $\mathscr{S}_t$, we define the eight-dimensional descriptor:

$$s_t = [s_t^{ns} s_t^{mb} s_t^{nls} s_t^{nrs} s_t^{lhb} s_t^{rhb} s_t^{mls} s_t^{mrs}] . \qquad (3.7)$$

Finally, re-identification based on skeletal features is performed by sorting distances of probe-cumulated skeleton descriptor with previously acquired cumulated descriptors of candidates.

3.3.5 Joint Face-Body Re-identification

Let us consider a sequence as a set $\mathcal{T}$ of ordered tuples $\mathbf{t}_t : \langle \mathbf{f}_t, \mathbf{s}_t \rangle$, where $\mathbf{f}_t$ is a face crop from the depth image and $\mathbf{s}_t$ is a set of skeletal joint feature defined in Sect. 3.3.4. Applying the COM to $\mathcal{T}$, we can obtain the cumulated model for face $\mathbf{f}$ and skeleton $\mathbf{s}$. To perform re-identification, let us consider a probe $\mathbf{t}_p := \langle \mathbf{f}_p, \mathbf{s}_p \rangle$. Re-identification is the task of sorting identities $\mathcal{I}$ in the gallery $\mathcal{G}$ by similarity with probe $\mathbf{t}_p$. We compute a distance for each identity $\mathcal{I}$ accumulating distances of every subsequence in the gallery:

$$D^f(\mathcal{I}, \mathbf{f}_p) = \sum_{i \in \mathcal{I}} d(\mathbf{f}_i, \mathbf{f}_p) \cdot \mathrm{rank}^f(i) , \qquad (3.8)$$

and for skeletons

$$D^s(\mathcal{I}, \mathbf{s}_p) = \sum_{i \in \mathcal{I}} d(\mathbf{s}_i, \mathbf{s}_p) \cdot \mathrm{rank}^s(i) , \qquad (3.9)$$

where i is a sample of identity $\mathcal{I}$, and $\mathrm{rank}^f(i)$ and $\mathrm{rank}^s(i)$ are rank of sample i according to face and skeleton feature distance.

We compute the final identity ranking using:

$$D(\mathcal{I}, \mathbf{s}_p, \mathbf{t}_p) = \alpha D^f(\mathcal{I}) + (1 - \alpha) D^s(\mathcal{I}) , \qquad (3.10)$$

where we set $\alpha = 0.6$ considering the better performance of face alone (this value has been determined on a preliminary set of experiments on a small set of training data).

3.4 Experimental Results

We test both our algorithms with dataset we have collected and released.

3.4.1 Datasets

We collected two datasets, a dataset of hand imagery named 'MICC Hand Pose,' since no other such dataset exists and 'Florence 3D Re-Id,' a novel dataset of people performing natural gestures at varying distances from the sensor.

The hand pose dataset consists of 18,188 and 15,937 RGB-D pairs of images of, respectively, open and closed hands, from nine different subjects. RGB-D pairs are synchronized and extracted at distances from 1 to 3 m from the sensor. Subjects recorded sequences both with sleeves rolled up and sleeves rolled down in order to avoid bias in the dataset. A sample of processed hands taken from our dataset is shown in Fig. 3.7.

Many previously collected datasets picture unnatural motions, such as standing still in front of the camera, or walking in circle. We instruct subjects to move in front of the sensor varying their distance, in order to capture biometric cues in different conditions. We also allow and encourage subjects to perform any task they are willing to do, such as reading their watch, interacting with a smartphone, or answering a call. All these actions are performed without any time line or choreography. Figure 3.1 shows two sample frames from our dataset, highlighting challenging situations that can happen in the case either the quality of the acquisition for skeleton or face data are low. So, our dataset includes strong variations in terms of distance from the sensor, pose, and occlusions.

We record three separate sequences for each of the 16 subjects included in the dataset. The first two sequences contain different behaviors performed standing. The third sequence of each subject pictures a sit-down and stand-up sequence in order to analyze the criticality of skeletal representation for non-standing poses. In particular, in this latter case, the joints estimation provided by the Kinect camera is more critical due to self-occlusions. Potentially, more stable solutions for occluded joints estimation could be used [25]. We collect depth frames at a 512×424 resolution (Kinect 2 standard) and the skeleton estimation with joint state (tracked/estimated). We also collect, but do not use in this work, face landmarks and the 3D face model fitted by the Microsoft SDK.[2]

The dataset is comprised of 39315 frames. Skeletons are acquired in 17982 frames, while faces are captured at a distance suitable for reconstruction (0.5–1.5 m) in 2471 frames.

Re-identification experiments have been performed separately for face and skeleton, and for their fusion. In the following, we first summarize the datasets used and then report on the obtained results.

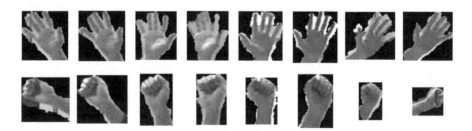

Fig. 3.7 Pose and orientation variation

[2]The Florence 3D Re-Id dataset is released for public use at the following link http://www.micc.unifi.it/.....

Hand Pose Recognition Results

We trained our system on eight subjects and report the accuracy on one kept out for testing; we trained the system on 31,172 (16,728 open and 14,444 closed) images and tested on the remaining 2,953. Without the use of temporal smoothing, the system achieves fairly accurate results with an overall accuracy of 96.34%. We improved the preliminary results by almost 10% by enlarging the dataset with around 20 k images. Moreover, care was taken in introducing all sources of variability in the data: rotation, scale, hand size, and clothing. The use of temporal smoothing increased the accuracy further, raising it to 98.95%. In Fig. 3.8, we show the classifier accuracy (after temporal smoothing) as a function of the distance of the subject from the sensor. These results clearly indicate that, within a distance of 3 m from the camera, results are extremely stable. Figure 3.9a shows the main sources of classifier errors. These are mainly due to low contrast images like frames (a) and (b) or a wrong segmentation as in frames (c)–(e). All but one of these errors are removed by temporal smoothing. The classifier error in frame (e) is recoverable by increasing the filter inertia as can be seen in the black box in 3.9b.

Smoothing did not impair system responsiveness; as shown in Fig. 3.9b, the transition of the detector (continuous red line) happens in just two frames and closely follows the transition of the ground truth. Increasing filter inertia (higher σ) can filter some erroneous predictions as seen in the black box, but this comes at the cost of a less prompt transition (see transition region marked by the arrow). Transition time is measured as the number of frames needed for the detector to switch from an open (closed) to a closed (open) state. Transition times are 2, 5, and 10 frames, respectively, for $\sigma = 10^{-3}, 10^{-2}$, and 10^{-1}, as shown in Fig. 3.10. Considering that our system runs at around 20 frames per second, the transition always happens in less than a second, while with the use of persistence in order to obtain a reliable input the timing is usually on the order of seconds (3s for XBOX 360 applications).

Our system runs at around 20 FPS on a 2.8 GHz core i7 CPU using a single core. Most of this computation time is spent in tracking and detection, while feature computation has almost no impact on performance. The use of a nonlinear kernel in the classifier negatively affects the testing time. This issue can be addressed with explicit

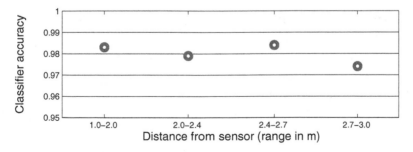

Fig. 3.8 Accuracy at various distances

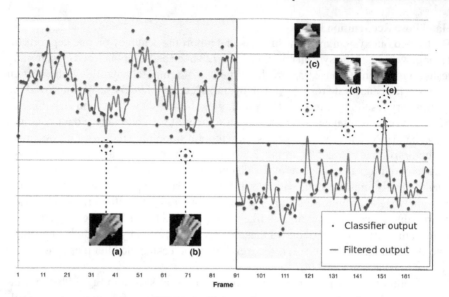

Fig. 3.9 Effects of temporal smoothing

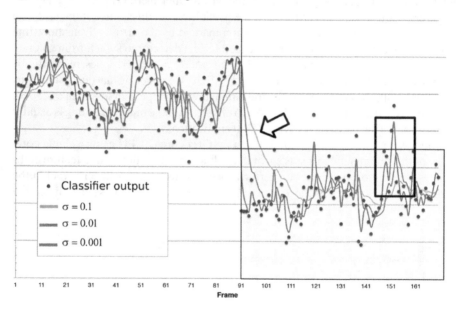

Fig. 3.10 Trade-off between responsiveness and accuracy

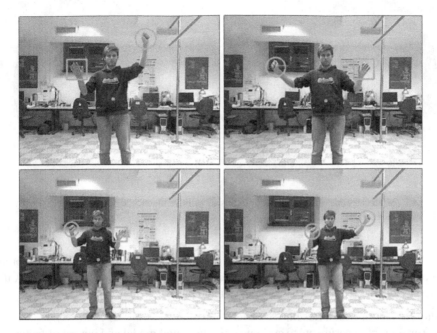

Fig. 3.11 Hand status detection: square (open hand) and circle (closed hand)

feature mapping in order to use linear classifiers that do not require the comparison of the test pattern with all support vectors.

In Fig. 3.11, four sample frames of the running system are shown. The system can handle multiple people, but for clarity of presentation we show frames with a single user. Note how the hand status recognition is invariant with respect to rotation, arm pose, background, and distance from the sensor. Videos of the system running are available online.[3,4]

Face Re-identification Results
In this experiment, we performed re-identification by using the models of the face reconstructed using full sequences and subsequences with 300, 200, and 100 frames, respectively. In this way, we can evaluate the behavior of our model on sequences with different number of frames and observe how this impacts on the selection of 'good' frames for reconstruction. This behavior can be visually appreciated in Fig. 3.12, where some reconstruction examples using the full sequence and sequences with 300, 200, and 100 frames are reported. It can be noted, there is quite a large variability in the quality of the reconstructed models in the case only part of the sequence is used, and in general the perceived visual quality improves with the number of frames.

---

[3]http://vimeo.com/38687694.
[4]http://vimeo.com/38687794.

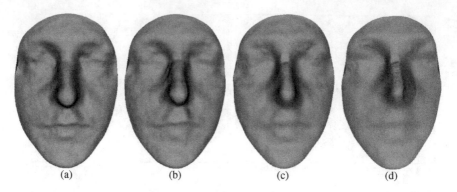

(a)   (b)   (c)   (d)

Fig. 3.12 Models reconstructed for one subject using: **a** full sequence; **b** 300 frames; **c** 200 frames; **d** 100 frames

For comparing reconstructed face models, the face description and matching approach proposed in [23] has been used. Results are reported in Table 3.2. Quite evidently, it emerges the performance drop in using full and partial sequences.

Body Re-identification Results

We run a set of experiments to evaluate our cumulated model and our set of features for re-identification. We vary the time frame over which recognition is performed. We show in Table 3.3 the difference between the weighted and unweighted model. The use of Eq. (3.3) to weight skeleton features allows better recognition rate. Clearly, the larger the set of skeletons influencing the final descriptor the better the recognition. On full sequences, weighting skeleton quality allows an improvement of 7% in recognition accuracy, which is much more than for shorter sequences. This is motivated by the fact that in longer sequences there is a higher chance of finding highly unreliable skeletons, which if unweighted will drastically worsen the performance.

Evaluation Of Body-Face Re-identification

Finally, we report the CMC curves on subsequences of different length evaluating our fused model exploiting skeleton and face re-identification jointly. In Fig. 3.13, we report CMC for different subsequence length. In the ideal case of full sequences, the

Table 3.2 Re-identification true acceptance rate (TAR) using face models reconstructed on sequences with different number of frames

	#probes	TAR (%)
Full sequences	32	93.8
Subsequences 300 frames	75	65.3
Subsequences 200 frames	87	56.3
Subsequences 100 frames	106	56.6

Table 3.3 Rank-1 recognition rate varying time frame constant τ, using Eq. (3.3) (weighted) or not (unweighted)

Sequence length	Weighted	Unweighted
Full sequence	**41.7**	34.7
Subsequences 300	**31.3**	30.2
Subsequences 200	**31.0**	30.1
Subsequences 100	**28.7**	27.9

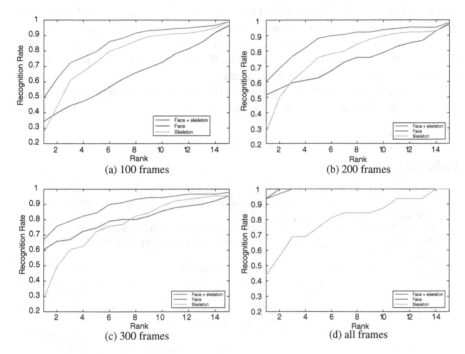

Fig. 3.13 CMC for fusion model on 100, 200, 300, and full sequences. The fusion model helps especially on short subsequences

use of skeleton does not add much to the almost perfect recognition we obtain from super-resolved faces, with a rank-1 recognition rate of 93.8%. In more realistic scenarios, when less frames are available, it can be seen that the fusion of the two features is extremely valuable. Indeed, faces have always a better rank-1 recognition rate, but the fusion model scores always higher than face and skeleton alone, raising rank-1 accuracy too.

3.5   Conclusions

This chapter presented two effective solutions based on RGB-D imagery. Hand status recognition is possible up to 5 m; nonetheless, existing trackers cannot reliably provide hand imagery at that distance. In the range 1–3 m, we have responsive and extremely accurate results that allow user interface to be deployed based on the proposed technique.

Furthermore, we presented a method for re-identification designed for RGB-D sensors. We show how super-resolved faces, with a cumulated observed model, can be used to recognize people very effectively. We also present an analogous strategy to cumulate observations of skeletons. Recognition using skeletal data is less effective, although is more applicable at a distance. Finally, our fusion model outperforms both single cue methods on short realistic sequences.

Both these modules have been integrated into working prototypes improving the functionalities and immersivity of the approach.

References

1. Bagdanov AD, Del Bimbo A, Seidenari L, Usai L (2012) Real-time hand status recognition from RGB-D imagery. In: Proceedings of ICPR, pp 2456–2459
2. Bondi E, Pala P, Seidenari L, Berretti S, Del Bimbo A (2016) Long term person re-identification from depth cameras using facial and skeleton data. In: Proceedings of UHA3DS workshop in conjunction with ICPR
3. Alon J, Athitsos V, Yuan Q, Sclaroff S (2009) A unified framework for gesture recognition and spatiotemporal gesture segmentation. IEEE Trans Pattern Anal Mach Intell 31(9):1685–1699
4. Ferracani A, Pezzatini D, Del Bimbo A (2014) A natural and immersive virtual interface for the surgical safety checklist training. In: Proceedings of the 2014 ACM international workshop on serious games. 2014 ACM Inc. pp 27–32. https://doi.org/10.1145/2656719.2656725
5. Oikonomidis I, Kyriazis N, Argyros A (2011) Efficient model-based 3D tracking of hand articulations using kinect. In: Proceedings of the 22nd British machine vision conference
6. Suryanarayan P, Subramanian A, Mandalapu D (2010) Dynamic hand pose recognition using depth data. In: Proceedings of ICPR
7. Ren Z, Yuan J, Zhang Z (2011) Robust hand gesture recognition based on finger earth mover's. In: Proceedings of ACM MM
8. Zheng WS, Gong S, Xiang T (2011) Person re-identification by probabilistic relative distance comparison. In: IEEE conference on computer vision and pattern recognition (CVPR). Colorado Springs, CO, USA, pp 649–656
9. Lisanti G, Masi I, Bagdanov A, Del Bimbo A (2015) Person re-identification by iterative reweighted sparse ranking. IEEE Trans Pattern Anal Mach Intell 37(8):1629–1642
10. Lisanti G, Masi I, Bagdanov A, Del Bimbo A (2015) Person re-identification by iterative reweighted sparse ranking. IEEE Trans Pattern Anal Mach Intell 37(8):1629–1642
11. Barbosa BI, Cristani M, Del Bue A, Bazzani L, Murino V (2012) Re-identification with RGB-D sensors. In: International workshop on re-identification in European conference on computer vision (ECCV) workshops and demonstrators. vol 7583, LNCS. Springer, Florence, Italy, pp 433–442
12. Pala F, Satta R, Fumera G, Roli F (2016) Multimodal person re-identification using RGB-D cameras. IEEE Trans Circuits Syst Video Technol 26(4):788–799

13. Satta R, Pala F, Fumera G, Roli F (2013) Real-time appearance-based person re-identification over multiple KinectTMcameras. In: International conference on computer vision theory and applications (VISAPP), pp 407–410
14. Baltieri D, Vezzani R, Cucchiara R (2014) Mapping appearance descriptors on 3D body models for people re-identification. Int J Comput Vis 111(3):345–364
15. Munaro M, Basso A, Fossati A, Gool LV, Menegatti E (2014) 3D Reconstruction of freely moving persons for re-identification with a depth sensor. In: IEEE international conference on robotics and automation (ICRA). Hong-Kong, pp 4512–4519
16. Shotton J, Fitzgibbon A, Cook M, Sharp T, Finocchio M, Moore R, Kipman A, Blake A (2011) Real-time human pose recognition in parts from a single depth image. In: Proceedings of CVPR
17. Lowe DG (2004) Distinctive image features from scale-invariant keypoints. Int J Comput Vis 60(2):91–110
18. Hu MK (1962) Visual pattern recognition by moment invariants. Trans Inf Theory 8:179–187
19. Bay H, Ess A, Tuytelaars T, Van Gool L (2008) SURF: Speeded up robust features. Comput Vis Image Underst 110(3):346–359
20. Berretti S, Pala P, Del Bimbo A (2014) Face recognition by super-resolved 3D models from consumer depth cameras. IEEE Trans Inf Forensics Secur 9(9):1436–1449
21. Rusinkiewicz S, Levoy M (2001) Efficient variants of the ICP algorithm. In: Proceedings of international conference on 3D digital imaging and modeling (3DIM). Quebec City, Canada, pp 145–152
22. Ferrari C, Lisanti G, Berretti S, Del Bimbo A (2015) Dictionary learning based 3D morphable model construction for face recognition with varying expression and pose. In: International of Conference on 3D Vision (3DV). Lion, France, pp 509–517
23. Berretti S, Del Bimbo A, Pala P (2013) Sparse matching of salient facial curves for recognition of 3D faces with missing parts. IEEE Trans Inf Forensics Secur 8(2):374–389
24. Shotton J, Girshick R, Fitzgibbon A, Sharp T, Cook M, Finocchio M, Moore R, Kohli P, Criminisi A, Kipman A et al (2013) Efficient human pose estimation from single depth images. IEEE Trans Pattern Anal Mach Intell 35(12):2821–2840
25. Rafi U, Gall J, Leibe B (2015) A semantic occlusion model for human pose estimation from a single depth image. In: IEEE conference on computer vision and pattern recognition workshops (CVPRW), pp 67–74

Chapter 4
Case Studies: BLSD and Surgical Checklist

Abstract In this Chapter, we describe the design and development of low-cost solutions, exploiting Microsoft Kinect ™ and 3D graphics, for two specific use cases: the simulation of the Basic Life Support Defibrillation (BLSD-S) and Surgical Safety Checklist (SSC-S) procedures. These prototypes have been designed with the aim to propose innovative pedagogical models. The main goal is to provide trainees with realistic activities to be performed during the simulation that must then be reproduced in the real experience. Gamification techniques and role-playing are used to engage trainees with well-defined roles of medical teams. The systems can be easily set-up and deployed in different spatial arrangements (part of this chapter previously appeared in Ferracani et al. (Proceedings of the 2014 ACM international workshop on serious games. ACM Inc., pp 27–32, 2014 [1]) ©2014 Association for Computing Machinery, Inc. Reprinted by permission; and in Ferracani et al. (Univ Access Inf Soc 14(3):351–362, 2015 [2]) with permission of Springer.).

Keywords Case studies · Immersive environments · Virtual reality · Emergency medicine

4.1 Introduction

Two immersive simulators (BLSD-S and SSC-S) provided with 3D graphics and natural interaction capabilities have been designed and developed in collaboration with healthcare professionals, in particular first aid experts for the BLSD-S and surgeons and their assistants for the SSC-S. The aim of these simulators is to train decisional skills of medical operators and to improve performance in carrying out standard security procedures through the immersivity provided by the realism of the virtual 3D scenario and the engagement with the system that natural interfaces are well known to improve. Both prototypes use paradigms of interaction borrowed from serious gaming in order to further engage users with the system. User performance is measured producing reports of simulation sessions, recording data about execution time, and errors committed by players. The two prototypes can run on every standard

© The Author(s) 2017

A. Del Bimbo et al., *Natural Interaction in Medical Training*, SpringerBriefs in Human-Computer Interaction, https://doi.org/10.1007/978-3-319-61036-8_4

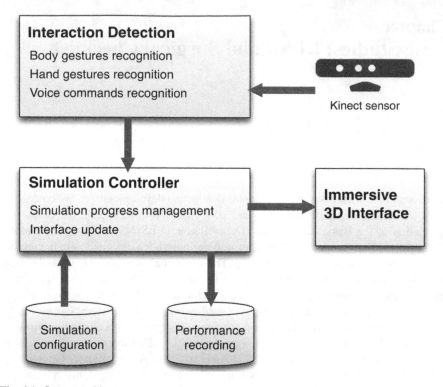

Fig. 4.1 System architecture

PC and use a Kinect sensor™ to detect user's interactions. A demo video of both systems is available online.[1]

The general architecture of the systems is presented in Fig. 4.1. Users' position and movements are tracked through the RGB and depth cameras of the Kinect while the Kinect's embedded array of microphones is used to detect voice commands. Information from the sensor are elaborated by an interaction detection module. In particular, the module is able to detect:

- **Body gestures** Using the Microsoft Kinect™ APIs[2], the position and orientation of all the skeleton's joints of the user is tracked in real time. A set of simple body gestures that users can perform to control the avatar, such as walking, rotating, and bending has been defined for the BLSD-S. For each gesture, ad hoc classifiers and Finite-State Machines algorithms which rely on skeleton joints position, translations, and rotations have been implemented to determine whether the user is performing a specific gesture required in the simulation. As an example, in the BLSD-S, the user can control the current view and walking direction of the avatar

---

[1] https://vimeo.com/124400550.

[2] http://www.microsoft.com/en-us/kinectforwindows/.

turning his torso; a Finite-State Machine algorithm for detecting this rotation tracks the position of user's shoulders, spine, and torso in order to observe a change in the user's orientation relative to the sensor.

- **Hand gestures** Some phases of the simulation require the user to perform hand gestures in both scenarios. This could be the case when the user is interacting with some virtual 3D object or when he is required to select options form virtual menus. Users can perform hand gestures such as pointing, pushing, or grabbing along with a swipe gesture that is used to activate a contextual menu in the SSC-S to interact with the simulations.
- **Voice commands** The SSC-S simulation is specifically designed to train communication skills and requires verbal interactions between team members or between a team member and the patient. In this scenario, users exploit their voice to control the virtual simulation. The Microsoft Speech SDK[3] is used to detect voice commands, converting voice into text that is then elaborated by the Simulation Controller module. Furthermore, since the Kinect sensor features an array of four separate microphones, the direction from which the voice is coming is determined by comparing each microphone response to the signal. This information is used to understand which user is speaking in the SSC-S multi-user scenario.

The Simulation Controller receives information about user interactions and, based on the current state of the simulation, produces the adequate visual feedback on the 3D interface. This module is also responsible for recording the simulation activity of each user, such as time spent in carrying out tasks and number of errors, information that is used by medical instructors to assess the performance of trainees. Instructors can create different simulation configurations for each session, changing environmental variables and clinical condition of the patient in both scenarios. Virtual environments of the two prototypes are based on the Unity3D [3] game engine and can run on any recent hardware. Scenes and models have been created with Maya.

4.2 BLSD-S Simulator Prototype

The BLSD simulator prototype (BLSD-S) is a 'serious' game developed in the context of the RIMSI project.[4] The simulator was designed as a single-user application which could be used to train medical personnel in the *Basic Life Support with Defibrillator* or BLSD procedure. Basic Life Support with Defibrillator is a procedure of medical care used for victims of life-threatening injuries or illnesses that can be provided by trained medical personnel, emergency medical technicians, paramedics, and qualified bystanders in the immediacy of the event until patients can be given full medical care at a hospital. The sequence of steps for the assessment and treatment

---

[3]https://msdn.microsoft.com/en-us/library/hh362873(v=office.14).aspx.

[4]Integrated Research of Simulation Models for the validation of processes and prototypes in surgical and emergency medicine, funded by Regione Toscana–Italy.

of the unresponsive victim have been defined and adapted to the virtual simulation with the help of first aid specialists following guidelines and recommendations
published in several states by associations and councils.[5] Generally, the procedures
span from ensuring the safeness of the environment where the BLSD is taking place
and assessing the patient level of consciousness to more advance treatments such
as early Cardiopulmonary Resuscitation (CPR), Automated External Defibrillator
(AED), and post resuscitation care.

The prototype follows the principles of the so-called 'serious' games technologies
for the improvement of skills and knowledge in medical activities. Serious games are
designed for a primary purpose other than pure entertainment. Furthermore, systems
featuring virtual reality and natural interaction can provide an highly interactive environment where students and teachers can improve learning with respect to standard
learning methods and applications. This is especially true if users can embody and
control their virtual representations (or avatars), making them closely react to their
actions, in realistic simulations. Currently, most of the simulated training sessions
in medicine occur in real environments such as laboratories, though more realistic
digital simulations that facilitate learning in a safe environment can be implemented
through these emerging technologies which exploit tracking and VR 3D graphics.
The BLSD-S provides a 3D virtual environment, high-resolution graphics and a
natural interaction interface to improve the effectiveness of the training of medical
personnel in first aid emergency situations. The prototype provides an immersive
and smart digital environment which can respond to natural gestures and actions of
team members in a simulated scenario. The system has been developed to improve
the learning methods currently in use and to solve some of their common issues such
as the poor memorability of procedures and the low efficiency in time execution.

BLSD-S simulates a first aid scenario and provides a virtual environment that
can be configured through an editor using interactive 3D objects and graphics. The
prototype is designed as a free roaming game, where the trainee can guide his virtual
avatar in the 3D environment to interact with virtual objects and the patient. The goal
is to complete a BLSD procedure in an indoor situation with potential environmental
risks for the operator and the patient (e.g., a gas leak). The user interacts with the
simulation through a natural interface using body gestures such as walking, rotating
or bending, or with hand gestures to select options in virtual menus. Gestures are
detected analyzing depth data obtained from the Kinect™ sensor without the need of
wearing additional hardware. This improves the immersivity of the system. A pre-
hospital scenario with several critical environmental arrangements, customisable by
instructors through an editor, has been selected and pre-configured for the simulator
since these emergency situations are the most expensive and difficult to reproduce
in simulation facilities.

In order to evaluate the prototype, several heuristics have been chosen and tested
to measure the overall system usability (see Sect. 4.2.7). A quantitative evaluation has
also been conducted analyzing outcomes of trainees, trained or not with the BLSD-S,
in carrying out standard procedures in Sect. 4.2.8. Results show that systems adopting

---

[5]More at Wikipedia: https://goo.gl/zx21aS.

natural interaction in immersive virtual environments and exploiting principles of serious gaming receive good feedback from users and improve their performance.

4.2.1 The BLSD Procedure

The Basic Life Support and Defibrillation (BLSD) procedure is a first aid technique based on the guidelines published by the European Resuscitation Council.[6] The BLSD is a procedure that can be accomplished by anyone who knows it and not necessarily by an healthcare operator. The goal is that of saving a person in danger of life even before the intervention of emergency professionals. The BLSD procedure can be performed by a rescuer once he have realized that there is a patient with a possible cardiac arrest and he has already called for help and Advanced Life Support (ALS). The main steps of the procedure are the following:

1. **Evaluation of the scenario and of the environmental safety**. Before starting the emergency procedure on the patient, it is necessary to assess the presence of any environmental hazards such as fire, flammable or toxic gas, exposed electrical cables.
2. **Assessment of the subject's state of consciousness**. The emergency operator must be on the left side of the patient laid possibly on the ground, on a rigid surface. To assess the state of consciousness, the operator calls him aloud and shakes him, trying to wake him up with vocal and manual solicitations. In the case the patient is not conscious, the operator continues with the BLSD.
3. **Opening of the airways and oral cavity inspection**. In case of presence of foreign bodies in the oral cavity these should be removed to avoid a cardiac arrest (e.g., movable prostheses, food residues, toys). In the presence of liquids, the operator must try to facilitate their leakage by tilting the patient's head. Subsequently, airway opening maneuvers must be performed to prevent the tongue from obstructing the oral cavity: I. Hyperextension of the head: The operator places the palm of the hand on the patient's forehead and slightly pushes the head back. II. The operator raises the chin of the patient with the other hand pointing upwards. In case of a cervical trauma, the hyperextension procedure must not be performed.
4. **Assessment of respiratory activity**. Keeping patient's head in the extended position the operator approaches the cheek to the victim's mouth and verifies the presence of respiratory activity. At the same time, he observes the movements of the chest. This procedure is known as 'Look, Listen, and Feel': The operator watches the movements of the chest, he listens if there is any respiratory noises, he feels the hot air coming out of the mouth of the victim on his cheek. The procedure must be done for about 10 s. If the patient does not breathe, the heart massage should be started.

---

[6]https://www.erc.edu/.

5. **External Heart Massage (CPR Cardiopulmonary Resuscitation)**. The cardiac massage is a chest compression technique that rhythmically applied stimulates blood circulation and avoids brain anoxia. To perform a correct heart massage, the operator must kneel next to the chest of the victim, on the left side, with the leg at his shoulder height. The patient's chest should be naked to be able to verify the correct position of the hands. The palm of the first hand should be placed in the middle of the chest, on the lower half of the sternum. The base of the palm of the other hand should be placed on the first one, and the fingers of both hands should be interwoven to secure that the pressure is on the sternum. The compressions should be made with arms stretched vertically at 90 o on the chest of the victim. The compressions should be performed at a speed of at least 100 compressions per minute (i.e., at least 3 every two seconds) by lowering the sternum by at least 5 cm. After 30 compressions, two ventilations should be performed and the procedure repeated five times.

6. **Assisted pulmonary ventilation**. The two lung ventilations can be carried out either by means of an appropriate instrument (called Ambu) or by mouth-to-mouth breathing. In mouth breathing, the operator with one hand closes the nose of the patient while with the other hand keeps the head in hyperextension pushing up the patient's jaw. Then the operator blows the air twice inside the patient's mouth. The puff should not be too energetic as there is a risk of hyperventilation resulting in an excessive increase in intrathoracic pressure.

7. **Cardiac rhythm evaluation and heart defibrillation (AED Automated External Defibrillator)**. The regularity of the heart rhythm is not assessed by the operator directly but through the use of the automatic external defibrillator (AED). Ventricular fibrillation as well as ventricular tachycardia can be the cause of a cardiac arrest. The defibrillation electric shock allows in such cases to re-synchronize the activity of the heart resuming its pump function and proper circulation. Defibrillators can be manual (usable only by medical personnel) or semiautomatic (can be used by non-health personnel). Fully automatic AED models exist that deliver the electric shock automatically without an activation by the operator. To perform the defibrillation, the operator must follow a precise procedure: (1) turn on the AED; (2) apply the electrodes: one beneath the right clavicle of the patient, the other below the left breast area along the front axillary line. This placements of the electrodes allows the defibrillation current to cross an amount of the myocardium as wide as possible; (3) at this point, the AED analyzes the rhythm and, if necessary, invites the operator to activate the shock; (4) the operator activates the shock and immediately removes the hands from the patient. If the AED recommends the operator not delivering the shock, the cardiopulmonary Resuscitation (CPR) should be resumed immediately waiting to run a new analysis of the cardiac rhythm or the arrival of professional healthcare staff.

4.2.2 The Scenario

In this chapter, one of the possible scenarios that BLSD-S prototype can simulate is presented: a Basic Life Support and Defibrillation (BLSD) procedure that has to be carried out by operators in a house with a gas leak. In this scenario, a player (the doctor) and an NPC (a first aid assistant) are used. Two of the provided avatar models are shown in Fig. 4.2.

This scenario depicts a typical BLSD procedure with the added risk of a gas leak. The gas smell and the possible leak are reported by the assistant. The player has to decide how to confront this situation: he could ask for help, leave the house, or locate the gas source. The player can move in the virtual rooms to check the environmental safety. If the player decides to locate the gas source and block the leak, then he can proceed to the BLSD procedure since putting safety into the environment is one of the prerequisites before getting care of the patient. An animation of the player removing the source of danger, in this case the gas leak, is used to signal that the procedure can start safely, as shown in Fig. 4.3.

Errors are reported by the medical assistant with audio and textual feedback. Timers are used in order to assess the player's performance and to consider the need of different procedures. To finalize the procedure, the player has to carry out certain actions in a specific order as shown by the flow diagram in Fig. 4.4. The BLSD procedure presented in Sect. 4.2.1 has been simplified in agreement and following the suggestions of first aid emergency professionals, considering the difficulty of

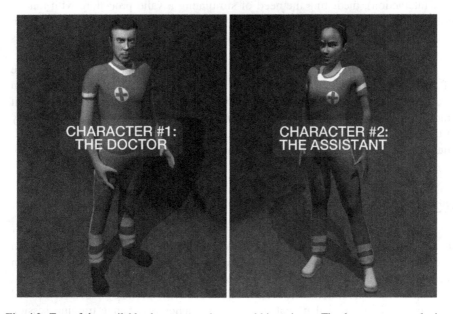

Fig. 4.2 Two of the available characters: a doctor and his assistant. The doctor acts as a playing character while the assistant as a NPC

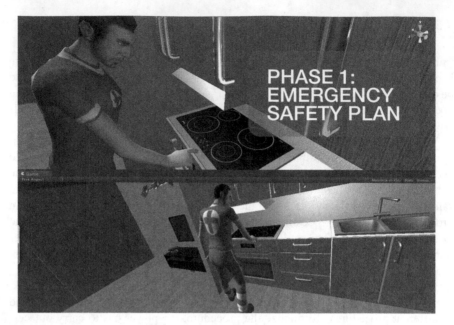

Fig. 4.3 Animation of player securing the environment before patient assistance

understanding and reproducing certain actions with the technology in use (e.g., natural interaction), mediating the need of simulating a valid procedure with that of obtaining a realistic natural interaction environment. These issues are analyzed in details in Sect. 4.2.4. A more evolved version of the prototype that partially solves these problems is presented in Sect. 4.2.9.

After securing the environment opening, the window the doctor has to take care of the patient, grab the proper tools, and activate them in the correct way. As an example, if a defibrillator is needed, the player has to catch it, turn it on, and wait until it is completely charged before activating it. The simulation ends successfully if the player completes the procedure correctly or unsuccessfully if he commits too many errors or delays in taking decisions. Some of these actions are shown in Fig. 4.5.

4.2.3   The System

The logical architecture of the system is shown in Fig. 4.6. The proposed system is composed by an immersive 3D virtual environment that allows user interaction through body gestures. Gestures are tracked using a Microsoft Kinect™ sensor and recognised by a dedicated software module. Furthermore, the system is composed by a configuration tool that enables medical teachers to change training session parameters as described in Sect. 4.2.5. Simulation sessions can be recorded in order

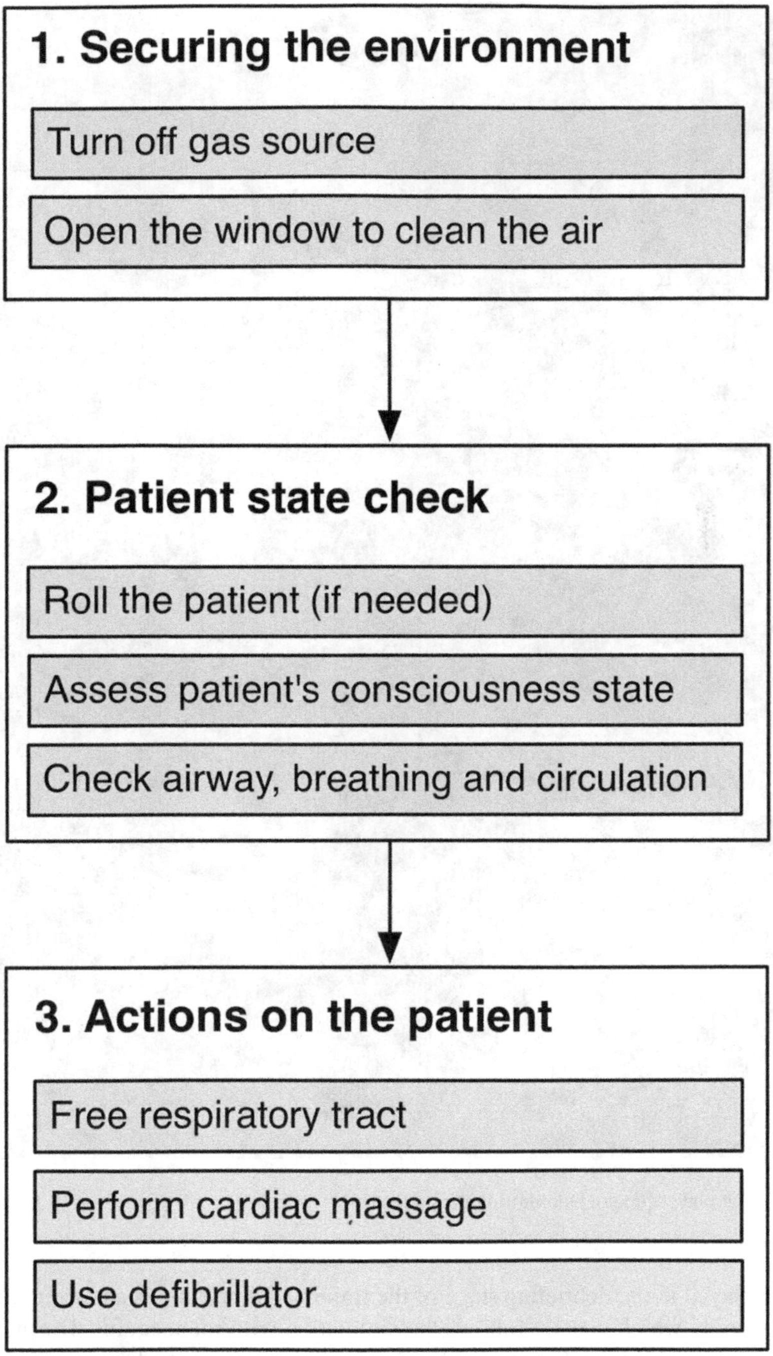

1. Securing the environment

> Turn off gas source

> Open the window to clean the air

2. Patient state check

> Roll the patient (if needed)

> Assess patient's consciousness state

> Check airway, breathing and circulation

3. Actions on the patient

> Free respiratory tract

> Perform cardiac massage

> Use defibrillator

Fig. 4.4 Correct sequence of the simulated BLSD scenario

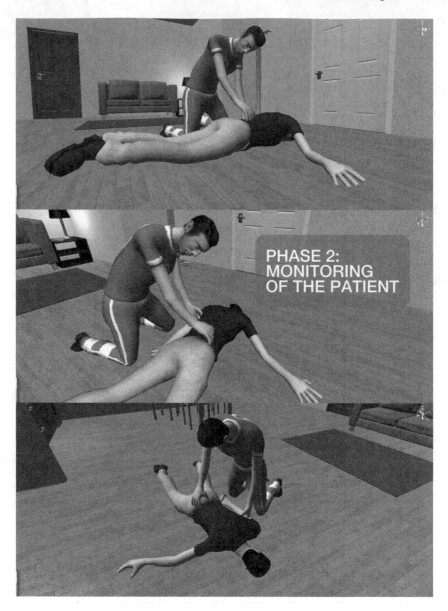

Fig. 4.5 The player (doctor) monitoring the patient

to be re-played in the debriefing stage of the training. Debriefing is an essential part of the training which usually follows the simulation with mannequins. During this phase, doctors and first aid operators discuss the circumstances and the actions taken by the team members in order to adapt the treatment, minimise errors, and to improve the performance of the overall procedure.

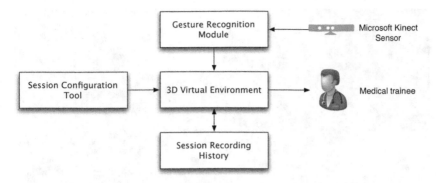

Fig. 4.6 Logical architecture of the overall system

In the following sections of this chapter, all the components of the system are described in detail.

4.2.3.1 Navigation and Virtual Environment

For virtual environments and natural interfaces to be effective, it is essential that the scenarios are realistic [4]. Consequently, all the environments, provided with forniture, where the BLSD procedure simulation takes place, as well as the avatars of the characters in the BLSD-S prototype have been designed and created with high realistic features. Some sample screenshots of this environment are shown in Fig. 4.7. Furthermore, avatars should be able to give realistic feedback also expressing emotions and reacting to natural *stimuli* so as to perceive as little as possible the distance between the digital representation of the characters and the real trainees. In this regard, mannequins can be quite realistic: in many medical simulation centers where, currently, simulator systems provided with mechanical patients are used, usually the trainee's task is to carry out some emergency actions on a mannequin whose vital signs are in the meantime monitored and controlled by training doctors present in another room. The trainees have the possibility to evaluate these parameters through a vital sign monitor. Their behaviors influence the responses and the reactions of the virtual patient, guided interactively by trainers. Though mannequins can be very realistic, as mentioned above, nevertheless laboratories equipped with high- and low-fidelity medical mannequins are expensive to build and to maintain while digital artifacts such as the BLSD-S allows to reduce organizational effort, to automate and increase the reproducibility and variability of training sessions, and to lower the cost of the staff required to manage the training.

In order to not underestimate the fact that a true realistic scenario requires the user to move freely in space and interact naturally with objects and persons, what happens in real life in the case of a simulation which uses mechanical patients, the BLSD-S simulator was designed as a free-roam game. A free-roam game is a game where there

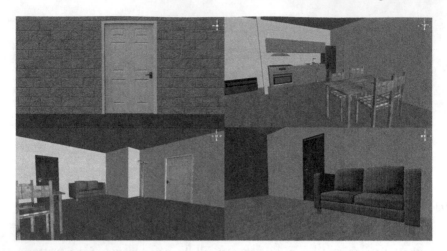

Fig. 4.7 A sample scene from the simulation prototype

is not a predefined order in which actions need to be executed in order to go on with the simulation and where the user can navigate the environment freely. This is obviously a mean of improving realism since, as in real life, a user may decide to take a direction rather than another, to assist a patient before another or to assess the environment safety before taking care of the patient. In order to fulfill this requirement allowing free navigation and interaction, the BLSD-S exploits natural interaction techniques through tracking and an ad hoc module, described in Sect. 4.2.4, which performs gesture recognition.

4.2.4 Gesture Recognition Module

The navigation in the BLSD-S virtual environment is made possible by a gesture-driven interface, which exploits the capabilities of the Kinect™, through which user behaviors are evaluated in order to interact with the scenario.

Simple or complex gestures can be recognized with the use of a depth camera and a skeletal tracking system [5]. Based on information extracted form, the depth and RGB cameras, the Microsoft Kinect™ APIs track the position and orientation parameters of all the joints of the skeleton model in real time. For every gesture that users can perform in the simulator, Finite-State Machine (FSM) models, FSM recognizers, and appropriate classifiers have been defined. In general, gesture recognition relies only on data from some specific body part, so for each gesture only significant skeleton joints are considered. Defined gestures can be found in Table 4.1, along with details about analyzed skeleton joints and consequent actions and behaviors performed by the virtual character.

Table 4.1 Association between gestures and character actions

Gesture	Body pose	Actions
Take/Grab	One of the hands moves in front of the body (on Z axes), an hand pose classifier has been implemented (see Chap. 3)	The character grabs objects in front of him/her, opens/closes handles
Rotate	The rotation of the torso is evaluated using x, y values of users' shoulders through FSM	The camera view of the person controller rotates in order to explore the scene
Walk-in-place	Sequences of x, y values of legs' joints are evaluated to check several phases of the walk through FSM	The character moves along the direction he/she is facing
Bend	Sequences of decreasing y values of chest and knees are evaluated through FSM	The character bends on his/her knees to examine the patient
Point	User's hand is in front of the body. x, y values are normalized with respect to the user's position in order to detect the gesture through FSM	A cursor is visualized in order to allow multiple choices

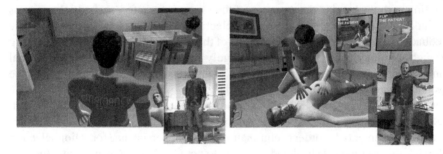

Fig. 4.8 Avatars performing actions based on the basis of user's gestures. In the bottom picture, a virtual menu with multiple options is shown

Gestures have been defined according to the requirements of the simulation context trying to allow users to interact in the virtual environment as they would do in real life. Simple actions and behaviors can be easily translated in natural body gestures or poses exploiting joints tracking provided by the Microsoft Kinect™ and Finite-State Machine algorithms. As examples, the rotation of the torso of the user in the simulation environment causes a rotation of the avatar and a change in the point of view in the virtual space, while the action of bending is used to approach the patient and check his condition and vital signs.

However, not each phase of the BLSD medical procedure can be associated with natural gestures due to the lack and the coarseness of the data from the Microsoft Kinect™ sensor that in some cases does not provide useful information to understand the situation and the actions performed by trainees. In fact, the lack of data such as the position of the fingers of the trainee and its low accuracy due to the complexity of the procedure step or person occlusions make impossibile to carry out in a natural way, for example the 'ABC procedure' (Airway, Breathing, Circulation) that has to be undertaken when the patient is unresponsive or unconscious. In the ABC, the first thing that has to be assessed is the smoothness of airway circulation which includes to verify the presence of airway obstructions caused by fractures of head and neck bones or foreign objects. Breathing assessment expects to check the good functioning of the lungs, chest wall, and diaphragm, and is evaluated by means of the 'Look, Listen, and Feel' procedure in order to see whether the patient breathes listening and feeling his breath. Finally, the trainee has to assess circulation of the patient by checking the pulse. If the pulse is palpable but the patient is not breathing, respiratory assistance can be given, whereas if the patient doesn't have pulse, 'Cardiopulmonary Resuscitation' (CPR) is needed.

When the trainee has to face a situation like the ABC, and eventually CPR, which is complex and implies a choice between different options and in a certain order, virtual menus appear in the BLSD-S simulation to allow the player to choose the action to perform. Figure 4.8 shows some of these phases of the interaction. Choices are presented as a list of thumbnails which depict the action to be performed accompanied by an explanation in textual labels. Items can be activated using persistence, i.e., pointing with the hand in the direction of the element for a few seconds. A progress bar indicating the time remaining before selection is shown below the thumb to give feedback to the user. Despite the unlikeness of this scenario in the real world, choosing through pointing an object is a paradigm largely known to players familiar with virtual games and digital simulations and it has shown little impact on the usability of the system as long as a good feedback and design are provided in order to illustrate these paradigms. Nevertheless, in a more advanced stage of prototype development, a classification algorithm for the recognition of the hand pose, described in Chap. 3, has been implemented in order to eliminate the need of persistence for action selection allowing the user to close his hands in order to activate items. Once an item (action) of the procedure is activated, feedback is given through virtual panels and, at the same time, if the trainee makes the right choice, an animation representing the action to be performed is played on the virtual avatar trying in this way to diminish the effect of 'loss of empathy' and engagement with the system caused by the interruption of the naturalness of the interaction flow.

4.2.5 Session Configuration Tool

In order to allow the instructor to change some aspects of the simulated scenario, a tool was developed to configure the training session. Through the use of this tool (shown in Fig. 4.9), trainers can change several parameters of the configuration and set up different scenarios. The tool allows trainers to place the patient in custom positions in the environment, to vary the environment itself and to add to each scenario several additional threats for the safety of patients and medical operators. Furthermore, it

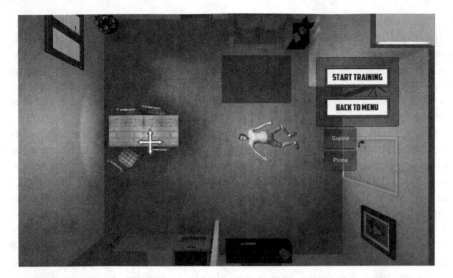

Fig. 4.9 Session configuration tool

is possible to simulate several patients conditions, adjusting the pose and the state of consciousness of the patient, and responses to therapies that require standardized procedures. In this way, the system can be useful even for multiple session, in order to assess trainee's behaviors in several situations. It is also possible to employ Non-Playable Characters (NPCs). NPCs are fictional characters not controllable by the player that provide predetermined and responsive behavior. In the BLSD-S simulator, NPCs can have different roles: They may be relatives, friends of the patient, or simple bystanders, they can also be members of the medical team performing the procedure. In both cases, they are employed to deliver information to the player. As a special case, an NPC can serve to augment the sensory input of the experience. As an example, although smell generators exist [6] and can be relatively affordable, an NPC can be exploited to provide information on the environment such claiming she is smelling smoke or other odors that may indicate danger. The use of the session configuration tool enables trainers to define complex and varied situations to keep trainees always engaged with the environment, and attentive to patient condition, and bystanders behaviors. The whole standard procedure can thus be learned as a complex interaction of medics, bystanders, and patients in the environment.

4.2.6 Assessment of Trainee Learning

In the BLSD-S prototype, the learning of trainees is assessed in two ways: (1) during the simulation through game dynamics and after the simulation measuring user performance (2) in a debriefing stage with instructors. During gameplay, the player is given continuous feedback from the system on the effectiveness of his/her actions using several audio visual and textual indicators (errors reported by the medical assistant, time elapsed, visual feedback to actions). Counting number of errors and measuring the time spent in carrying out tasks are part of the serious gaming mechanisms that induce the users to try to improve their performance stimulating the competition between trainees, also considering that the learning outcome is recorded and it is performed in group and in public in front of the other learners.

An important stage for medical training both in classic and new learning methods is the so-called 'debriefing'. Debriefing is an important method of learning for improving performance and the learning itself from committed errors during the simulation. Debriefing can be defined as a dialogue between two or more people; the main goals of it are to discuss the actions and processes involved in a particular patient care situation, stimulate reflection on those thought processes and actions, and incorporate improvement into future performance. In this concern, the function of debriefing is to understand aspects of team performance that went well, and those that did not. The discussion can be really important on determining opportunities for the improvement of the procedures at the individual, team, and system level.

In emergency medicine, debriefing in simulation is considered as important as the simulation itself [7]. In a real classic training session scenario, the debriefing usually follows the interactive simulation with mannequins. Debriefing is carried out to understand if the actions taken during the simulation and the interactions with the patient have been performed in a safe and correct way. During the debriefing, the trainers and the team of trainees discuss actions and mistakes often with the aid of a video record of the whole session: This is the stage where trainees learn more. The traditional debriefing classrooms have a teacher-centered approach, because trainees involved in the interaction session are not able to 'see' themselves and their errors. Moreover, in training sessions mediated by mannequins, users undergo behaviors and reactions. In natural interaction systems instead, individual responsibility, represented by the avatar or character in the game, and self-assessment are more relevant. In this sense, the BLSD-S uses a learner-centered teaching approach: The trainee is the user himself, through interaction, to guide the learning process resulting in a better memorability of the procedure. Furthermore, as a general rule it should be noted that, as shown by Villneuve et al., digital natives prefer the use of technology in learning [8].

In this respect, the BLSD-S not only allows the simulation of otherwise too expensive or dangerous situations but also greatly improves this phase of the training. Interactive sessions with the BLSD-S can also be re-played and used as training materials. The use of a completely virtual simulation also allows to produce digital logs of all the events occurring during the procedure and also virtually reproduce the situation during the debriefing. The game logs not only contain the progress of patient vital signs, his symptoms, and reactions but also the actions, the exact position, and the posture of all the players involved in the simulation. With this data, it is possible to literally playback the whole simulation, switching the point of view in the 3D virtual environment (what it is impossible in a camera recording) and analyzing in detail the behavior of all the participants. In this way, a large database can be built quickly to evaluate errors and the most common difficulties of trainees. This data, in addition to increasing the effectiveness of training, can be useful to assess how well the simulation environment work and how it can be improved.

4.2.7 Heuristic Assessment of the BLSD-S Virtual Environment

According to Nielsen [9], there are four main ways to evaluate a user interface: (1) formally by some analysis technique; (2) automatically by a computerized procedure; (3) empirically by experiments with test users; and (4) heuristically by simply looking at the interface and passing judgment according to one's own opinion. On one hand, inspection-based methods generally use guidelines or checklists as criteria to point out usability problems, although deciding which guidelines are applicable to particular problems usually becomes more difficult as the number of guidelines grows. On the other hand, heuristic evaluation methods are quicker to use since they employ a limited set of design principles or heuristics. Since heuristic evaluation is quick, it is a cost-effective method and traps a high proportion of usability problems with 4–5 trained evaluators [10]. The heuristics used in the present study are derived from Nielsen's work and from previous results about virtual environment design principles [11]. Starting from the heuristics proposed by Sutcliffe, a subset of heuristics that suited to the nature of our BLSD-S virtual environment was selected. In particular, emphasis was given to heuristics for evaluating the interaction intuitiveness and system immersivity. The following heuristics were chosen:

H1 **Natural engagement**. Interaction should approach user expectation of interaction in the real world as far as possible. Ideally, the user should be unaware that the reality is virtual.

H2 **Compatibility with the user's task and domain**. The VE and behavior of objects should correspond as closely as possible to user expectation of real-world objects.

H3 **Natural expression of action**. The representation of the self/presence in the VE should allow the user to act and explore in a natural manner and not restrict normal physical actions.

H4 **Realistic feedback**. The effect of the user actions on virtual world objects should be immediately visible and conform to the laws of physics and the user's perceptual expectations.

H5 **Faithful viewpoints**. The visual representation of the virtual world should map to the user normal perception, and the viewpoint change by body movement should be rendered without delay.

H6 **Sense of presence**. The user's perception of engagement and being in a real world should be as natural as possible.

Ten evaluators (six of them researchers in the field of interactive systems and four medical operators in the field of emergency medicine) were asked to interact with the

Table 4.2 Results of the heuristic evaluation questionnaire. Rating are expressed on a 5-point scale

	Statement	Rating
H1a	The interactions with the environment were natural	3.6
H1b	The gestures which controlled movement through the environment were natural	3.9
H2	The behavior of the objects in the virtual environment was close to my expectation	3.6
H3a	User's representation in the VE act naturally	3
H3b	User's representation in the VE match my body movements	4.1
H4a	The effects of user's actions on virtual world objects are immediately visible	3.4
H4b	Virtual world objects conform to the laws of physics and the user's perceptual expectations	4.1
H5	Avatars are designed to convey user's viewpoint and activity	4.1
H6a	I was sufficiently involved in the VE experience	4.3
H6b	I was concentrated on the assigned tasks rather than on the mechanisms used to perform those tasks or activities	3.1

virtual environment. Evaluators were instructed how to interact with the system, and the task they were supposed to accomplish was described to them. In particular, the correct medical BLSD procedure was explained and they were asked to perform it in the virtual environment. Eventually, evaluators were requested to fill a questionnaire based on the proposed heuristics. The questionnaire consisted of 10 declarative statements, each one relative to the chosen heuristics. Evaluators rated these statements using a 5-point Likert scale, from 1 (strongly disagree) to 5 (strongly agree). Average results of the heuristic evaluation for each statement are reported in Table 4.2.

The results show that users were highly engaged in the virtual reality experience (H3b, H5, H6a), even though there are still some issues related to gesture understanding, interaction with objects, and tasks accomplishment (H2, H3a) whose concerns have been pointed out and partially solved in Sects. 4.2.3.1 and 3.2.

4.2.8 Usability Testing

To assess the validity of the BLSD-S system through a quantitative measurement of its usability in terms of educational enhancement, an evaluation has been conducted with a group of 26 students attending the last year of the medicine school and therefore already familiar with the correct medical procedure. The simulation scenario was defined with doctors in order to be performed both with the virtual interactive system and with the standard simulation method based on the use of an high-fidelity mannequin as a patient located in a dedicated and equipped room. Students were equally divided in two groups, group A and group B. Students from group A were

Table 4.3 Results of simulation of the two groups

	Group A	Group B
Avg. procedure time (s)	741	631
Avg. procedure correctness (%)	46	93

trained exclusively with the standard simulation approach, while students in group B performed a training session with the virtual interactive system before experiencing the standard simulation. Table 4.3 shows results in term of time and percentage of correct procedure steps achieved by students from the two groups during the standard simulation. Although a mannequin-based simulation allows to train a broader range of skills, results suggest that the use of the virtual simulation could effectively improve outcomes in the whole training process.

4.2.9 Improving Immersivity and Naturalness of Interaction of the BLSD-S

Some of the BLSD-S prototype limits emerged during its development as well as the availability on the market of new interaction sensors and more immersive virtual reality displays have led, in a second stage, to the implementation of an advanced BLSD-S (II) prototype. The new prototype provides a setting in which the trainee can play the simulation staying seated wearing an head-mounted display (i.e., the Oculus Rift). Navigation (i.e., locomotion) and interaction are allowed using only hand gestures through a Leap Motion. An idea of the arrangement of the simulation environment is given in Fig. 4.10.

The Oculus Rift[7] is a set of virtual-reality goggles that can be mounted on the head able to transport the user in a virtual space. This is accomplished using a pair of screens that displays two images side by side, one for each eye, which create a stereoscopic 3D image. This choice was made in order to further improve the results for some of the heuristic evaluation reported in Table 4.2. Heuristics in H4b, H5, and H6a though giving good outcomes still had room for improvement, especially in terms of 'Faithful viewpoints' and 'Sense of presence'.

More relevant were the problems related to the navigation and interaction emerged in the scenario described in the first prototype, in particular: (1) the difficulty of movement caused by the navigation modality in the environment. The user is forced to move his legs (through 'Walk-in-place', see Table 4.1) and at the same time to rotate his torso which, in addition to causing fatigue, sometimes results in errors. This is due in to the low accuracy of the action detection, which is complex, to the difficulty of control of the action itself on a virtual representation and to the

---

[7]https://www.oculus.com/rift/.

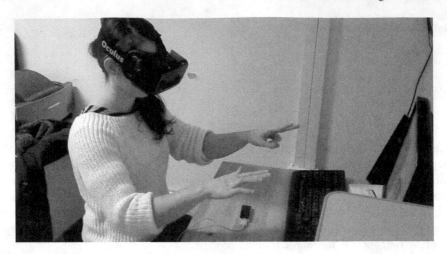

Fig. 4.10 A trainee during a simulation with the BLSD-S prototype exploiting the Oculus Rift and the Leap Motion controller

presence of obstacles in the virtual environment which force the users to continuous rotations, stops, and restarts for moving (see H1b heuristic in 4.2); (2) issues with the naturalness of interaction with 3D objects due to the limits of the Kinect sensors in terms of availability of data, precision, and occlusions. As noted in Sect. 4.2.4 and as emerged from the heuristic evaluation in Table 4.2, the overall naturalness of the system is not as good as you could expect. It is rated 3 in H3a and also rates relative to object interaction (H4a: 3.4), and naturalness of acting (H6b: 3.1) are not high. This is conceivably due to the fact that too complex actions and procedures in the BLSD-S scenario are replaced with metaphorical paradigms of interaction or virtual menus (i.e., in some phases of the 'ABC' Airway, Breathing, Circulation, and in the CPR 'Cardiopulmonary Resuscitation' procedures). To solve both of these issues, it was thought to use a sensor such as the Leap Motion that would allow: (1) the implementation of hand-based motion gestures for locomotion that would permit to relieve the fatigue of 'Walking-in-place'; (2) the detection of more precise and complex gestures and actions on the patient that would allow to remove virtual menus and make the user experience completely natural. The Leap Motion[8] is a sensor device that supports hand and finger motions as input, analogous to a mouse, but requires no hand contact or touching. The device consists of two cameras and three infrared LEDs. The cameras track infrared light with a wavelength of 850 nm, which is outside the visible light spectrum. The sensors are directed along the y-axis upward when the controller is in its standard operating position and have a field of view of about 150°. The Leap Motion controller provides information about hands and each finger on a hand. If all or part of a finger is not visible, the finger characteristics are estimated based on recent observations and the anatomical model

---

[8]https://www.leapmotion.com/.

of the hand. Furthermore, the Leap Motion SDK natively provides the recognition of some gestures (i.e., Swipe, Circle, Screen Tap, Key Tap) but still gives developers the ability to implement their own action recognition systems. Both native gestures and ad hoc recognition systems have been used in implementing the new prototype. On this basis and exploiting these technologies, some improvements to the BLSD-S were introduced and the experience redesigned trying to improve performance and overcome issues described above.

4.2.9.1 Simulation Scenario and Navigation

The simulation scenario is the same described in Sect. 4.2.2: a first aid intervention in a indoor environment where there is a gas leak and an unconscious patient lying on the floor. The trainee is seated at the simulation station, wearing an head-mounted display (i.e., the Oculus Rift) and can make gestures with hands that allow him to navigate and interact with the virtual environment. These gestures are tracked and detected by a Leap Motion sensor placed on a flat surface (a table) in front of the user, see Fig. 4.10. Unlike the first version of the scenario, the user experiences the virtual environment in first and not in third person. This choice has been made with the aim of increasing the degree of immersion of the system also considering the use of the Oculus Rift. To focus user attention to hand gestures and to increase even more the immersion of the system, the hands and part of the trainee's arms present in the field of vision of the trainee are reproduced in the simulation environment through some highly realistic models, available in the system, that are adapted at runtime to the physical measurements of the users (as an example see Fig. 4.11). In this way, the trainee has continuous feedback on the position of his hands, on the gestures made and on system responses and reactions.

Locomotion is enabled in this version of the BLSD-S prototype (II) exploiting the 'Screen Tap' gesture provided by the Leap Motion SDK. The user can start moving in the environment simply tapping in the air above the sensor and then heading the movement through the orientation of the hand. Tapping has been designed as a metaphorical gesture for locomotion consisting in a tap with the index finger in the direction the user wants to start walking. It is a gesture not so far from the real world: People commonly use the index finger to show a walking direction. This choice is based on the results of a study [12] we conducted on various interaction modalities for achieving the so-called infinite locomotion in immersive virtual environments through natural interaction. The study has highlighted how the 'Tap gesture' is perceived by users as natural as the traditional 'Walk-in-place' method that it provides a better precision and can be effective in alleviating fatigue-related issues, making interaction possible also staying seated. To stop moving, the user can simply perform a 'stop hand gesture' in the field of view of the Leap Motion as when you flash your palm at someone, in order to pause or stop him.

The simulation presents a subset of the possible procedures, described in Sect. 4.2.1, to be performed in the case of a BLSD intervention. The patient is in fact on the ground, unconscious and no response to CPR maneuvers is assumed.

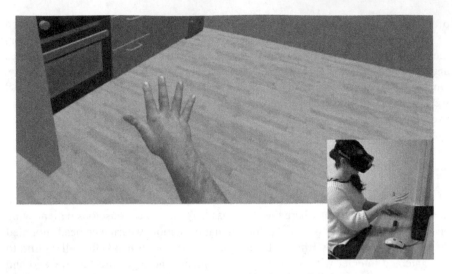

Fig. 4.11 Hand and forearm of the trainee reproduced in the virtual environment

Once in the indoor environment, the rescuer is in front of the patient which is unconscious due to a gas leak. An NPC's external voice warns the operator of the present danger (i.e., the gas leak). The first thing to do is therefore to secure the environment: first of all the, operator must close the gas knob, then open the window for the air exchange, and finally, take care of the victim, see Fig. 4.12(1–3). To do these actions, the trainee can use natural gestures that are detected by the Leap Motion sensor. However, in order to assist the user in correctly performing gestures, the system can also be configured in an assisted mode in which the gestures to be performed are presented and suggested through a semiopaque reproduction of the hands of the operator, as shown in Fig. 4.12. The suggestion of the hands position is triggered in the scenario contextually to the status of the procedure and only when needed as the user is close to certain objects (i.e., the gas knob and the window) or is taking care of the patient. It is especially useful for more complex actions: at the beginning of the simulation to allow the user to understand how to move in the environment (locomotion is allowed using 'Tap gesture' and then controlling the heading with the hand) or in case of advanced procedures to be performed on the patient, e.g., the hyperextension of the head in Fig. 4.12(6), CPR cardiac massage in Fig. 4.12(7), CPR lungs ventilation in Fig. 4.12(8), positioning of the electrodes in Fig. 4.12(9). The use of the assisted mode is particularly suitable for the first training of operators, the use of visual suggestions being primarily effective in increasing the memorability of the actions to be performed. Once the operator has secured the environment, he must assist the patient. First of all, in order to assess the consciousness of the patient he can try to stimulate a response through a slight slapping on his face, see Fig. 4.12(4). The 'slapping' is one of the gestures not provided by the Leap Motion sensor that has been implemented for the simulation. As the patient does not respond, the operator passes to inspect the airways, detecting the presence of a foreign body in the mouth that he can remove through a natural gesture, see Fig. 4.12(5). The contingency of a scenario with a gas leakage and at the same time an airway obstruction of a patient is rather unlikely, but it was created in order to emphasize one of the fundamental components of a proper BLSD procedure. In fact, to obstruct, the airway may also be the tongue itself of the victim or, in the case of elder people, their dental prostheses. Then the operator must perform the 'Look, Listen, and Feel' procedure which can only be carried out after the hyperextension of the patient's head, see Fig. 4.12(6). The hyperextension of the head expects that the rescuer places his right hand on the forehead of the patient while the index and medium fingers of the other hand exert an upward pressure under the chin. Since the patient doesn't breathe, the operator proceeds to CPR. The cardiac massage cannot be performed correctly in the simulation, because it would be very difficult to understand the position of the both hands one above the other through the depth sensor which is sensible to occlusions. So we chose to focus the attention of the trainee more on the number, the rhythm, and the sequence of compressions and ventilations. The user can perform compressions keeping both hands opened on the chest of the patient, see Fig. 4.12(7). A counter indicates when the user reaches thirty compressions. The synthesized voice of the NPC gives continuous feedback describing how well the trainee is performing (if he is going too slow or too fast) in addition to explaining the correct way to position the hands. The two lungs ventilations are executed tapping the nose of the patient with the right hand upholding his chin with the left hand in order to hold the head hyperextended, see Fig. 4.12(8). An animation simulates the zoomed view of the patient while the operator breathes mouth-to-mouth. The sequence is repeated for five times. In the last step of the procedure, the rescuer uses the AED. First, he must correctly place the electrodes whose position is suggested by the simulator (on the right below the clavicle, on the left below the chest). Once the AED has completed the heart rhythm analysis, it invites the operator to deliver the electric charge. The operator activates the button using the 'Screen Tap' gesture; see Figs. 4.12(9–10).

Finite-State Machine (FSM) recognizers are used for the detection of all the gestures implemented in this second version of the BLSD-S prototype unless gestures provided by the Leap Motion SDK are exploited. For locomotion, the built-in 'Screen Tap' gesture is used while heading is provided evaluating the normal of the fingers when the arm is stretched with the palm of the hand facing down (Fig. 4.11). 'Screen Tap' is also used to activate the electric shock delivered by the AED as described in Fig. 4.12(10). The other additional gestures implemented using FSM models instead are defined to be an ordered sequence of states in the spatial-temporal space. These states take into account mainly: (1) the position of hands and fingers in time and space; (2) the location of the hands and fingers with respect to the body of the patient; (3) the persistence of such positions in time according to predefined thresholds. Using these models, it is possible to describe and detect actions such as the grabbing and torsion of the hand used in Fig. 4.12(2, 4) for closing the gas knob and opening the window and special configurations of one or both hands such as slapping in order to check the state of consciousness, for freeing the respiratory tract, for head hyperextension, CPR cardiac massage, CPR lungs ventilation, and AED electrodes

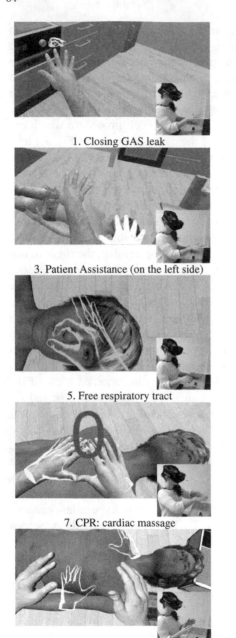

1. Closing GAS leak

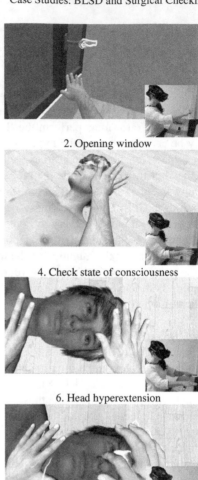

2. Opening window

3. Patient Assistance (on the left side)

4. Check state of consciousness

5. Free respiratory tract

6. Head hyperextension

7. CPR: cardiac massage

8. CPR: lungs ventilation

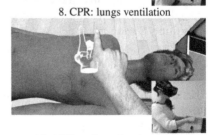

9. AED: place the electrodes

10. AED: activate the electric shock

Fig. 4.12 BLSD scenario procedure

placement, represented, respectively, in Fig. 4.12(4–9). In two cases, (i.e., 4. slapping to check state of consciousness and 7. CPR cardiac message) also the rhythm and speed of executions of the single actions which compose the sequences are considered analyzing data provided by the Leap sensor relative to the hand palm shift speed.

4.2.9.2 BLSD-S (II) Prototype Evaluation

The new version of the BLSD-S (II) prototype has been evaluated in two ways: (1) through a questionnaire to users whose questions assess interaction intuitiveness and system immersivity. The same heuristics in 4.2.7 proposed by Sutcliffe [11] exploited to evaluate the Kinect-based prototype were used. Results are compared; (2) through a comparative evaluation between the two versions of the BLSD-S (I-II) simulators which assess trainees learning of correct BLSD procedures (results obtained exploiting a questionnaire).

In Table 4.4, results of the heuristic evaluation between the two prototypes, BLSD-S (I) and BLSD-S (II), are shown.

The heuristics questionnaire was submitted to the same people which evaluated the first version of the prototype using the same questions. Results show that (1) the issue related to the difficulty of locomotion in the environment has been mitigated

Table 4.4 Comparison between the heuristic questionnaire for both prototypes. Rating are expressed on a 5-point scale

	Statement	Rating v. I	Rating v. II
H1a	The interactions with the environment were natural	3.6	3.8
H1b	The gestures which controlled movement through the environment were natural	3.9	4.5
H2	The behavior of the objects in the virtual environment was close to my expectation	3.6	3.8
H3a	User's representation in the VE acts naturally	3	4.5
H3b	User's representation in the VE matches my body movements	4.1	4.1
H4a	The effects of user's actions on virtual world objects are immediately visible	3.4	4.3
H4b	Virtual world objects conform to the laws of physics and the user's perceptual expectations	4.1	4
H5	Avatars are designed to convey user's viewpoint and activity	4.1	4.8
H6a	I was sufficiently involved in the VE experience	4.3	4.5
H6b	I was concentrated on the assigned tasks rather than on the mechanisms used to perform those tasks or activities	3.1	3.8

through the use of the new mechanism which adopts the 'Screen Tap' gesture in place of 'Walk-in-place' (H1b passed from 3.9 to 4.5); (2) the overall naturalness of interaction increased a lot in H3a from 3 up to 4.5 and also object interaction and naturalness of acting have been improved, respectively, from 3.4 to 4.3 (H4a) and from 3.1 to 3.8 (H6b). These results are plausibly due to the removal of virtual menus, to a greater proximity to the actual gestures to be made during the procedure allowed by the Leap motion and the gesture detection models and to the overall improved immersivity of the system obtained through the use of the Oculus Rift and the design of a first-person experience (see heuristics H3b, H5, H6a).

In order to assess and compare the learning outcomes of the training with both versions of the prototypes, a questionnaire with ten questions on some of the procedures of the BLSD has been submitted to two groups of 10 trainee. All the students were at the beginning of their university medical education and had no previous knowledge of the procedure. People in the two groups were randomized to reduce as much as possible bias mainly related to different familiarity with digital and VR technologies. As the two simulations were not perfectly comparable with regard to the steps of the procedure, proper voice feedback regarding these aspects has been added to the first prototype before testing (in fact, in the scenario presented with the BLSD (II) more advanced actions can be performed and details are presented such as how to execute the cardiac massage, how to position the hands for the hyperextension of the head, the number of compressions and ventilation in the CPR, the positioning of the AED electrodes.).

The questionnaire consists of 10 multiple choice questions. Some sample questions with answers are reported here: (1) what is the first thing to do in a BLSD scenario? (a: take care of the patient; **b: secure the environment**; c: none of the above options); (5) is the patient's breathing status to be checked before starting head hyperextension and eventually CPR? (**a: yes**; b: no; c: I do not know); (9) where have DAE's electrodes to be placed on the patient? (a: the first under the left clavicle and the second on the right side; **b: the first under the right clavicle and the second on the left side**; c: in none of the two previous positions). The average of correct answers for the group of students who had a training session with the BLSD (I) prototype, i.e., the Kinect-based one, was 80% while for students who did training with the BLSD (II), based on Oculus Rift and Leap Motion, was 87%. Hence, the new version seems to give better results in terms of knowledge gained by trainees with respect to the first version. This confirms how likelihood, naturalness, and immersion of the system through VR and natural interaction can improve the effectiveness of the training and improve learning.

4.3   SSC (Surgical Safety Checklist) Simulator Prototype

The SSC-S simulator prototype exploits natural interaction paradigms and realistic 3D interfaces in order to train doctors and students in the use and accomplishment of the Surgical Safety Checklist (SSC). The SSC is a medical procedure that has to be carried out before a surgical operation as defined by the World Health Organization[9] in order to minimize the risks endangering the lives of surgical patients. After the introduction of the Surgical Safety Checklist by the WHO, that has to be carried-out by surgical team members, several studies have proved that the adoption of this procedure can remarkably reduce the risk of surgical crisis.

The natural interface provides an interactive virtual environment that aims to train medical professionals in following the security procedures proposed by the WHO adopting a 'serious game' approach and exploiting virtual reality and natural inter-action as a mean of engagement with the training system. Serious games and virtual reality systems have been widely exploited in medicine training and rehabilitations. However, although many medical simulators exist with the aim to train personal skills of medical operators, only few of them take into account cooperation between team members and exploit natural interaction.

The system presents a realistic and immersive 3D interface and allows multiple users to interact using vocal input and hand gestures. The game can be seen as a role play game in which every trainee has to perform the correct steps of the checklist accordingly to his/her professional role in the medical team. A multiplayer game with turn and role-taking dynamics is resulted highly suitable in designing a simulator to train a medical team which need to collaborate in this task. The simulator associates users with a professional role on the basis of their position in the physical space (i.e., anesthesiologist, surgeon, and nurse) and reproduces the scenario which precedes a surgical operation. Focus groups and discussions with surgical teams have been conducted which have highlighted how the checklist can be and usually is performed by these three operators. Every step of the checklist requires one of the three operators to interact with the others or to check the status of medical devices. Voice-based interactions occur when one of the professionals is expected to communicate with the patient or with another team member. Hand gestures are used to check the state of the medical equipment or to activate virtual menus.

The virtual 3D simulation can be visualised on a large-sized screen or projection and users can interact with the virtual simulation using body or hand gestures as well as voice commands. To detect interaction of the users with the simulation the system use a Microsoft Kinect™ sensor. Compared to the BLSD-S (I) scenario, in which the user has to explore the virtual space, this second scenario is more static. The focus is on the training and the improvement of communication skills between the operators and the respect of roles and tasks to be accomplished. Natural interactions between users and the simulator are obtained exploiting the Microsoft Kinect ™ sensor which provides a layer on which gesture detection systems can be implemented and an SDK for performing voice recognition.

From a didactic point of view, the SSC-S simulator allows the trainers to observe the dynamics of dialogue between the trainees and the trainees to familiarize natu-rally with the procedure. Sessions are re-playable and can be reused effectively in the debriefing phase where committed errors, role exchanges, insecurities can be analyzed and discussed.

---

[9]http://bit.ly/1fHMDZm.

The system is easily deployable requiring only a standard PC, a projector and a Kinect sensor.

4.3.1 Surgical Checklist

The SSC-S is part of the so-called vocational training systems where the need is to train an activity which is usual in the everyday job of surgeons. Surgical-care is a central part of health care throughout the world, counting an estimated 234 million operations performed every year [13]. Although surgeries are essential to improve patients health conditions, they may lead to considerable risks and complications. In 2009, the World Health Organization[10] (WHO) published a set of guidelines and best practices in order to reduce surgical complications and to enhance team work cooperation [14]. The WHO summarized many of these recommendations in the Surgical Safety Checklist, shown in Fig. 4.13. Starting form the proposed guidelines, many hospitals have implemented their own version of the SSC in order to better match requirements of internal procedures.

The SSC identifies three main distinct phases corresponding to a specific period during the execution of an operation: 'before the induction of anesthesia,' 'before the incision of the skin,' 'before the patient leaves the operating room.' In each phase, the surgical team has to complete the listed tasks before it proceeds with the procedure. All the actions must be verified by a checklist coordinator who is in charge to guarantee the correctness of the procedure. The goal is to ensure patient safety checking machinery state and patient conditions, verifying that all the staff members are identifiable and accountable, avoiding errors in patient identity, site, and type of procedure. In this way, risks endangering the well-being of surgical patients can be efficiently minimized.

Gawande et al. [15] conducted several simulations of a surgical crisis scenario in order to assess the benefits obtained by the adoption of the SSC. Results have shown that the execution of the SSC improves medical team's performance and that failure to adhere to best practices during a surgical crisis is remarkably reduced.

The WHO recommends that all system and method implemented in order to carrying out the procedure meets three main objective of the procedure itself: (1) 'does the entire team stop all other activity for a few moments at three critical points, i.e., pre-anesthesia, pre-incision, and before the patient leaves the OR? The goal is for the entire team to participate in each pause. (the surgeon may not have to be present for the pre-anesthesia check.)'; (2) 'Does the entire team verbally confirm each item on the WHO Checklist? The goal is for the entire team to participate. At a minimum, every item on the WHO Checklist should be confirmed. Other items may also be addressed'; (3) 'Are the items verified without reliance on memory? The goal

---

[10]http://www.who.int/.

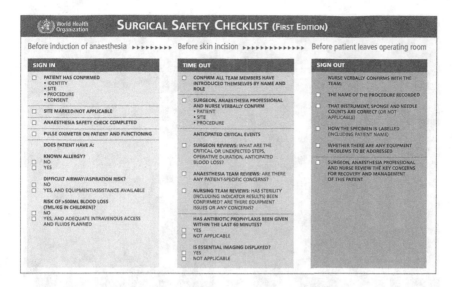

Fig. 4.13 The surgical safety checklist proposed by the WHO in 2009

is to use a tool for reference to ensure every item is covered, e.g., a form, poster, or computer screen.'[11]

The proposed system is a serious game featuring an immersive virtual environment (IVE) to train and practice users in the accomplishment of the surgical checklist. The SSC-S adopts natural interaction via gestures and voice. The system acts de facto as the 'checklist coordinator' of the surgical team. The simulation involves multiple trainees (up to three), each of them associated with his/her role, and guides them throughout a complete SSC procedure in a surgical operation scenario. The three actors (the surgeon, the anesthesiologist, and the nurse), expected to complete the checklist, are automatically detected by the system when approaching the IVE and can interact gesturing and speaking as in the real life. Interactions and choices are not mediated by haptic devices or other controllers but mimic how the real procedure should be conducted.

4.3.1.1   Simulation Scenario

The virtual simulation allows the three health professionals who are going to execute a surgical operation to complete the SSC, with respect of their professional role. The IVE was designed with the objective to help the trainees to understand the correct procedures to be followed. Professionals (i.e., trainees) stand in front of the simulation interface (see Fig. 4.14). The simulator associate users with a professional role on the basis of their position in the physical space. The interface provides at the

---

[11] http://www.who.int/patientsafety/safesurgery/checklist_implementation/.

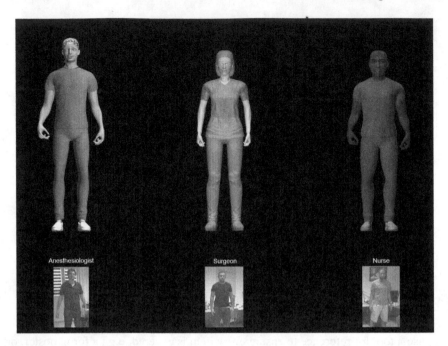

Fig. 4.14 Avatar selection: the trainee can choose which role to enact standing on the left, on the center, or on the right of the IVE

bottom of the application view an RGB representation of the space in which the simulation is taking place captured through an RGB camera which is set up in axis with the depth sensor (i.e., the Microsoft Kinect™). This RGB view is divided in three part giving feedback to users to where to place themselves in the space to enact the proper role (anesthesiologist, surgeon or nurse, see Fig. 4.14). In practice, the user standing on left will be associated with the anesthesiologist, the one in the center will be the surgeon, and the trainee on the right will be the nurse. These RGB camera views of the trainees are present during all the scenes and the entire session of the simulation. In this way, the trainee can always verify his position in the space, check if he is recognized by the system as the active user or not (an iconic representation of the operator on the left of each RGB camera view container lights up when the correspondent user is considered 'active'), and see himself interacting, as shown in Figs. 4.15 and 4.16.

Once each user is associated with a role, the IVE is shown and the simulation can start. The first environment represents the pre-operating room, where usually the 'before the induction of anesthesia' phase of the SSC takes place, with the patient laying on the bed and the three professionals' avatars around him. From this moment, the trainee can take control of the simulation by taking a step ahead. When one of the user has control, the environment is shown from his/her first-person point of view

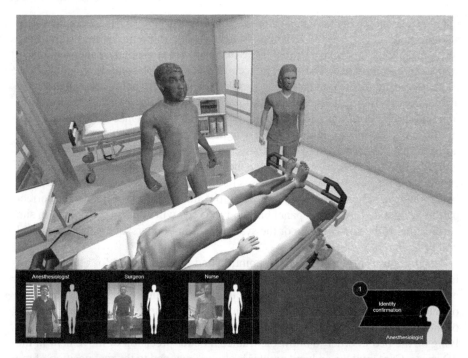

Fig. 4.15 A 3D pre-operating room environment from a first-person POV, showing the patient and other professionals' avatars

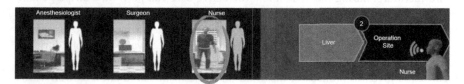

Fig. 4.16 The second step of the procedure, the nurse must confirm the operation site

(POV), see Fig. 4.15. Hence, the active user can interact via voice or gesture in order to carry out the specific step of the SSC procedure.

Interactions can be performed both by voice or hand gestures. Voice-based interactions are used during the SSC when one of the professionals is expected to communicate with the patient or with another team's member in order to perform the procedure. For instance, one step of the SSC simulation contemplates that the nurse confirms to other team members the site of the operation they are going to do, let's imagine it to be the liver. Accordingly, the user enacting, the nurse should take a step ahead and say something like 'we are going to operate the liver' or a similar sentence. As soon as the sentence is pronounced, the system verifies if the site of the operation is correct (as explained in Sect. 4.3.3), it updates the SSC status, and it gives feedback in order to continue with the simulation. System feedback and suggestions on how to interact are given in the right side of the bottom bar where RGB camera views are also presented. Here, there's an arrow- shaped panel where the current step of the SSC procedure is reported in textual form. In the top left angle of the panel, a numeric stepper is also provided. The panel is accompanied by a placeholder figure for the character of the medical team that has to do that particular action and is currently active (e.g., the nurse is in charge to ask the patient and have a confirmation from him and the medical team that he must operate the liver). Once the user is active (in this case, the nurse), the placeholder figure is substituted with an image of the nurse avatar. An animation of sound waves emerging from the mouth of the figure indicates that the system is waiting for the voice input of the operator (if a voice command is expected). If the nurse poses the question 'are we going to operate the liver?' then the system analyzes the speech input and verifies if the liver is the correct part to be operated. A further panel blinking in green will confirm the operation site verification, if the site is wrong or the system does not understand instead the panel will blink in red, see Fig. 4.16.

Hand gestures instead (e.g., hand pointing and push) are used for other types of interaction, such as to touch the patient, to check the state of the medical equipment, or to activate virtual menus. Let's give another example: in the 'before the induction of anesthesia' part of the procedure, the nurse has to indicate with her hand the part of the body to be operated. The IVE displays the patient with a view from above lying on the bed in order to allow the trainee a better precision of movement in the 3D space. Contextually, an hand pointer is shown, mapped to the real position of the nurse's hand, which allows her to select the body part as shown in Fig. 4.17.

Furthermore, during the simulation, the active user can perform a *swipe* gesture with his hand to activate a virtual panel, shown in overlay, that contains all the information about the patient clinic history and the status of the SSC to be carried out. The overlay simulates the patient's medical card, always available during a real surgical operation. When all the steps of the checklist are correctly performed, feedback is given to trainees of the good outcome of the simulation as well as the report of the time spent in completing the procedure and the recording of all the errors committed by the user. The system exploits these data in order to provide the simulation with some gaming aspects: (1) The team members share the goal to correctly complete the checklist in the shortest time (the system provides a ranking table of the best team scores); (2) each trainee competes with the other team members, and his performance is measured by a scoring system which keeps track of all the individual errors and show the results at the end of the simulation.

Although the SSC have been strictly defined and formalized by the WHO at an high level, the 'content' of the simulation sessions is fully configurable in the system (i.e., the patient's anamnesis and clinic card: demographic infos, type of disease and surgery, allergies, instrumentation status, operational critics, postoperative treatment). This means that instructors can simulate, and trainees experience, all possible operations, risks, and patient's conditions. Therefore, different and more domain-specific scenarios can be created for teams of medical professionals in every field.

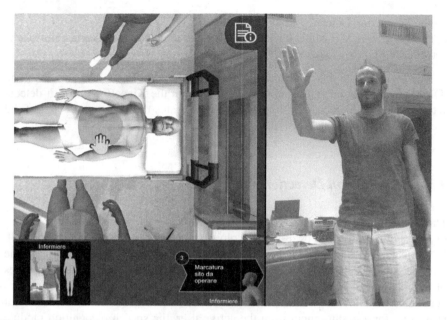

Fig. 4.17 The nurse indicates the patient's body part to be operated pointing his/her hand

The SSC-S interface has been designed keeping always in mind the three require-ments pointed out by the WHO and reported in Sect. 4.3.1: (1) the three critical points of the procedure, i.e., 'pre-anesthesia,' 'pre-incision,' and 'before the patient leaves the operating room' are covered by three different virtual scenes connected through animations. Each member of the team has to be present in each phase; (2) the entire team confirms each item of the checklist signing digitally the checklist itself at the end of the simulation; (3) the prototype doesn't allows to skip steps and the simulation can't go on if each action has not been performed correctly by the operator responsible of it. Furthermore, the session is logged in order to be verified by an automated system so that there is certainty that all checklist steps have been carried out correctly without errors.

4.3.2   The System

The proposed simulation system (the SSC-S) is a natural interface that exploits a realistic 3D interface and natural interaction paradigms in order to train users to correctly execute the SSC. Users stand in front of an large-sized screen or projection and can interact without using any wearable or hand-held device. Contrariwise they can use their voice and body as interface controller. The system is composed by two main modules:

- The Interaction Detection Module (IDM);
- The Immersive Virtual 3D Interface (IVE), and the associated Game Status Controller (GSC).

The logical system architecture has been presented in Fig. 4.1 in Sect. 4.1: The IDM analyzes motion and depth data coming from the Kinect™ sensor, it detects actions, and communicates with the GSC that updates the IVE on the basis of the scenario's configuration.

4.3.3 Interaction Detection

The interaction between users and the IVE is obtained tracking movements and identifying actions performed by users by exploiting the Microsoft Kinect™ sensor [16]. In particular, the interface can be controlled by trainees using their position in the physical space, hand gestures and voice (see Fig. 4.18). The three different types of interaction can be executed concurrently, or can be turned off/on by the system depending on the phase of the simulated procedure. For instance, if the simulator is waiting for a gesture input from the active user, the speech recognition module is temporarily switched off. The IDM is responsible of recognizing the actions and notifying them to the GSC module in order to proceed with the simulation.

In details, the IDM is able to detect:

- **Active user**. The Kinect sensor v. 1, used in the implementation of the SSC-S prototype, is able to identify up to six human figures standing in front of the camera, but it can only track two skeletons (with all their joints) simultaneously. Since the system is designed for three users and it is essential to be able to track the gestures and the position of the user hands, a policy is needed to dynamically define which of them is controlling the simulation (i.e., the interface). From the depth map obtained by the sensor, the IDM detects which user is closer to the interface. When a trainee performs one step ahead, resulting in a reduction of the

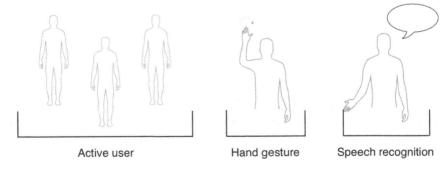

Active user   Hand gesture   Speech recognition

Fig. 4.18 Different types of interaction the system is able to detect

distance on the *z-axis*, the module notifies a change of the active user to the Game Status Controller. This detection is active during all the simulation session.

- **Hand gestures**. Once the active user is identified, skeleton tracking is exploited to detect his movements and, in particular, to track his hand position in the space. The hand position is used to map an hand pointer in the IVE used to interact with interface elements. The IDM tracks the active hand of the trainee and sends its spatial coordinates in the 3D space in order to update the interface. When the user needs to 'activate' some virtual element on the interface, he/she must perform a *push* gesture with the open hand. This is somehow similar to a *click* on a mouse-based interface. Hands tracking and gesture updates can be switched on/off by the GSC, depending on the phase of the simulation. Furthermore, a *swipe* gesture has been provided that allows the user to open a virtual 2D panel overlaid on the interface which reports the patient's case history and clinic card. This gesture is performed by moving the right arm from the right to the left in the field of view of the Microsoft Kinect™ sensor.

- **Speech inputs**. The Kinect features an array of four separate microphones spread out linearly at the bottom of the sensor. Data perceived by these microphones are analyzed in order to control the interface through voice commands. Furthermore, by comparing each microphone response to the same audio signal, the microphone array can be exploited to determine the direction from which the signal is coming and therefore to pay more attention to the specific sound in that direction rather than in another. The module checks if the angle from where the vocal input is detected corresponds to the position where the active user is, in order to ignore unexpected speech form other users. So, when the IDM has identified the active user, it tries to understand his/her specific audio signal. In order to achieve this, background noise removal algorithms are applied [17]. The Microsoft Speech SDK is used to verify the the correctness of trainees' questions and answers when interacting via voice with the system. In particular, it is exploited to asses whether user's vocal input corresponds to a correct value for the current SSC step.

In order to perform speech recognition a speech input, a speech recognition engine and a grammar are required. A speech grammar consists of a structured list of rules that identify words and phrases that the system should attempt to identify in the spoken input. Grammar rules can be simple word commands, such as 'Yes' or 'No,' but also more complex sentences such as 'It is correct that you must operate the liver?'. Rules define patterns and word sequences to be matched against the vocal input. Rules and patterns are described in an XML-format grammar that conforms to the Microsoft Speech Recognition Grammar Specification (SRGS) Version 1.0. Through grammars, a limited vocabulary in a certain domain can be defined so that a user is able to accomplish a specific tasks using the system only by speaking. Furthermore, grammars must be flexible and allow slight variations in spoken input to enable natural interaction and to provide a better user experience. For example, in the scenario of the SSC, the system must accept multiple ways that the trainee ask for patient identification: 'Are you Mario Rossi?', 'Is Mario Rossi your name?', 'We are going to operate Mario Rossi.' The Game Status Controller (GSC) dynamically loads the grammar (the scenario configuration file) which contains sets of possible keywords and phrases that are correct for the current step. Based on these sets, the module checks the audio input and computes a confidence value for the 'speech-to-text' match. If the detected confidence is greater than a threshold value, the correct interaction is notified to the GSC and the simulation can continue to the next step. Acoustic models, lexicons, and language models are used to search the best match of the input with the textual instances present in the grammar.

4.3.4 Game Status Controller

The Game Status Controller is the module responsible of the logic behind the whole simulation system. On simulation start-up, the controller parses the external Scenario Configuration file containing all the phases, possible questions, and correct answers for the current training session. On the basis of the configuration, the system initializes the 3D interface setting up the environment (e.g., the pre-operating room), the characters graphic appearance and all the information required (e.g., the information in the panel which contains the clinical history of the patient and the in-memory representation of all the procedure correctly performed). For each simulation phase and SSC procedure step, the GSC communicates to the IDM which type of interaction must be detected. In case of vocal input, the controller also evaluates the set of correct phrases to be recognised in the current phase of the simulation. The GSC receives interaction information and uses them to verify if the actions are correct or wrong according to the Scenario Configuration and the SSC. The controller then updates the interface in order to give positive/negative feedback to trainees and, consequently, to trigger animations and 3D cameras/points-of-view changes. All the actions and errors are recorded and stored in order to provide teams' and trainee's with performance feedback.

4.3.5 Implementation Details

The system is composed of two modules: the GSC/IVE and the IDM. The GSC module and the 3D immersive interface are developed within the Unity3D[12] environment using both C# and JavaScript programming languages for the interactivity. The Scenario Configuration file containing the SSC procedure structure and the patient case history and clinic card is in JSON syntax. The IDM which exploits Microsoft Kinect™ to detect users's interactions is developed in C# language and uses a network socket to communicate with the main program (the VR interface). Scenes and characters have been created using Autodesk Maya. The system can run on every normal Windows-based workstation and is easily deployable requiring only

---

[12]http://unity3d.com/.

to set up a Kinect sensor in front of the three trainees. The workstation have to be equipped with also an RGB Webcam which is used in order to give trainee a view on their position in the space and to take proper position in the environment in order to enact their role (see Fig. 4.15).

4.3.6 Classification and Initial Assessment of the SSC-S Prototype

According to its functionalities, the developed system can be described and assessed using the taxonomy proposed by Wattanasoontorn et al., as shown in Table 4.5. Wattanasoontorn et al. extended the classification system defined by Rego et al. [18] who identified a taxonomy of criteria for the classification of serious games for health (application area, interaction technology, game interface, number of players, game genre, adaptability, progress monitoring, performance feedback, and game portability).

During the entire design and development process of the SSC-S prototype, medical professionals have been involved in order to reproduce scenarios and procedures that are highly compliant with real surgical operations. An evaluation of the system has been conducted with 10 students through a questionnaire using the same heuristics of the BLSD-S (I-II) prototypes [19] to assess the naturalness and immersivity of the virtual interface. Results are shown in Table 4.6.

Future work will include several assessments of the system exploiting advanced usability testing [20].

Table 4.5 System classification by functionality according to Wattanasoontorn's taxonomy

Functionality	Solution
Application area	Cognitive
Interaction technology	Microsoft kinect
Game interface	3D
Number of players	Multiplayer (up to three roles)
Game genre	Role play
Adaptability	No
Performance feedback	Yes
Progress monitoring	No
Game portability	Yes
Game engine	Unity 3D / Kinect SDK
Platform	PC
Game objective	Professionals training
Connectivity	No

Table 4.6 Results of the heuristic evaluation questionnaire. Rating are expressed on a 5-point scale

	Statement	Rating
H1a	The interactions with the environment were natural	2.5
H1b	The gestures which controlled movement through the environment were natural	3.7
H2	The behavior of the objects in the virtual environment was close to my expectation	3.2
H3a	User's representation in the VE act naturally	2
H3b	User's representation in the VE match my body movements	2.1
H4a	The effects of user's actions on virtual world objects are immediately visible	3.8
H4b	Virtual world objects conform to the laws of physics and the user's perceptual expectations	3.0
H5	Avatars are designed to convey user's viewpoint and activity	4.4
H6a	I was sufficiently involved in the VE experience	4.5
H6b	I was concentrated on the assigned tasks rather than on the mechanisms used to perform those tasks or activities	2.2

4.3.7 Long-Term Re-identification for the SSC-S

The Cumulative Observation Model for person re-identification presented in Sect. 3.3.1 has also been used and implemented recently in our systems in order to extend the functionalities of both the prototypes, i.e., the BLSD-S and the SSC-S simulators systems. In fact, being able to recognize a trainee across multiple sessions can really increase the perceived naturalness of the systems and further engage the trainee with the simulators. Re-identification is carried out using a method which relies on face geometry matching of reconstructed 3D face models (Sect. 3.3.3) in combination with a method based on body part geometry which computes similar distances between couples of joints of the user torso (Sect. 3.3.4). The model has been implemented in the simulators to work in real time and to be able to re-identify users on the fly and continuously over the time. Furthermore, the COM has allowed the implementation of a module for automatic user performance evaluation without the need for complicated user session authentication and matching procedures. On the other hand, in particular, for the SSC-S scenario, it allowed the removal of interface paradigms which had a negative impact on the naturalness of multi-user role-changing dynamics. In fact, in the initial scene, the SSC-S simulation implied each user to take place spatially in a particular region of the room to embody his role (i.e., anesthesiologist, surgeon, or nurse). With the introduction of the COM re-identification system, however, there is no longer a need for this procedure and users can move freely in space without almost any errors in role assignment. Furthermore, trainees are not required to take a step ahead in order to express the intention to perform an action but they can simply start speaking and the system is able to understand if the audio source is coming from the person-in-charge to complete the action. This is done checking the angle of origin of the audio source with respect to the position of the trainee in the space. Finally, a simple interface has been implemented for the integrated data model management to record the hospital personnel and associate their role before the beginning of the simulations. The program exposes an interface which guides the user through three steps: (1) the operator inserts his data in the program (i.e., the ID, name, surname, and role) through a form panel; (2) the program asks the trainee to frame his head in a camera view. Then, it reconstructs a 3D face model of the observed person through the depth sensor and extracts SIFT keypoints (through RGB camera) and facial curves in order to perform face recognition, as described in Sect. 3.3.3; (3) the program asks the trainee to stand up, frame his upper body (i.d. the torso) in the camera view and then it extracts features relative to body geometry building an eight-dimensional descriptor for skeleton re-identification (see Sect. 3.3.4). All these features are used by the Cumulative Observation Model, described in Sect. 3.3.5, in the BLSD-S and SSC-S simulators to identify trainees and their roles on the fly and let them carry out the simulation so as to interact as smoothly as possible with the interface and avoiding identification at each session.

References

1. Ferracani A, Pezzatini D, Del Bimbo A (2014) A natural and immersive virtual interface for the surgical safety checklist training. In: Proceedings of the 2014 ACM international workshop on serious games, 2014. ACM Inc., pp 27–32. https://doi.org/10.1145/2656719.2656725
2. Ferracani A, Pezzatini D, Seidenari L, Del Bimbo A (2015) Natural and virtual environments for the training of emergency medicine personnel. Univ Access Inf Soc 14(3):351–362 Springer
3. Unity 3d game engine (2013). http://www.unity3d.com
4. Lok B, Ferdig RE, Raij A, Johnsen K, Dickerson R, Coutts J, Stevens A, Lind DS (2006) Applying virtual reality in medical communication education: current findings and potential teaching and learning benefits of immersive virtual patients. Virtual Real 10(3):185–195 Springer- Verlag, London, UK
5. Shotton J, Sharp T, Kipman A, Fitzgibbon A, Finocchio M, Blake A, Cook M, Moore R (2013) Real-time human pose recognition in parts from single depth images. Commun ACM 56(1):116–124
6. Scentsciences corporation (2012). http://www.scentsciences.com
7. Crookall D (1992) Debriefing. Simul Gaming
8. Villeneuve M, MacDonald J (2006) Toward 2020: visions for nursing. Technical report, Canadian Nurses Association, Ottawa, Ontario, Canada
9. Nielsen J, Molich R (1990) Heuristic evaluation of user interfaces. In: Proceedings of the SIGCHI conference on human factors in computing systems. ACM
10. Nielsen J (1993) Usability engineering. Access Online via Elsevier
11. Sutcliffe A, Gault B (2004) Heuristic evaluation of virtual reality applications. Interact Comput 16(4):831–849
12. Ferracani A, Pezzatini D, Bianchini J, Biscini G, Del Bimbo A (2016) Locomotion by natural gestures for immersive virtual environments. In: Proceedings of the 1st international workshop on multimedia alternate realities (AltMM 2016). ACM, New York, NY, USA, pp 21–24. https://doi.org/10.1145/2983298.2983307

13. Weiser TG, Regenbogen SE, Thompson KD, Haynes AB, Lipsitz SR, Berry WR, Gawande AA (2008) An estimation of the global volume of surgery: a modelling strategy based on available data. Lancet 372(9633):139–44
14. Haynes AB, Weiser TG, Berry WR, Lipsitz SR, Breizat AH, Dellinger EP, Herbosa T, Joseph S, Kibatala PL, Lapitan MC, Merry AF (2009) A surgical safety checklist to reduce morbidity and mortality in a global population. New Engl J Med 360(5):491–499
15. Gawande AA, Arriaga AF (2013) A simulation-based trial of surgical-crisis checklists. New Eng J Med 368(15):1460
16. Zhang Z (2012) Microsoft kinect sensor and its effect. IEEE Multimed 19(2):4–10
17. Webb J, Ashley J (2012) Beginning kinect programming with the microsoft kinect SDK. Apress, 12 Jun 2012
18. PA Rego, P Moreira, L Reis (2010) Serious games for rehabilitation: a survey and a classification towards a taxonomy. In: 5th Iberian conference on information systems and technologies (CISTI), pp 1–6
19. Sutcliffe A, Gault B (2004) Heuristic evaluation of virtual reality applications. Interact Comput 16(4):831–49
20. Bowman DA, Gabbard JL, Hix D (2002) A survey of usability evaluation in virtual environments: classification and comparison of methods. Presence Teleoperators Virtual Environ 11(4):404–24

Chapter 5
Conclusions

Abstract In this short book we have presented two prototype systems based on Virtual Reality and Natural Interaction born from a collaboration with doctors and professionals in the healthcare sector. Strong requirements by medical staff were the implementation of multimedia systems that could reduce training costs, facilitate task execution through automated procedures, reduce instrumentation and systems setup time and, above all, to improve trainee learning both in terms of refining individual skills and team collaboration. To these ends the BLSD-S and SSC-S were created.

Nowadays, medical simulation is an essential part of the training of doctors and medical practitioners. While simulation in its simplest forms has been adopted for centuries, the digital era has opened the doors for novel and more effective simulation methods. Fully virtual simulators with 3D graphic and intuitive interaction (both with haptic devices or gesture tracking) have been standardized, and their effectiveness has been evaluated in studies in several medical fields.

Initial skepticism in the adoption of such systems, mainly due to poorly realistic 3D graphic or high cost of visualization and tracking devices, has been quickly overcome in latest years. Since the early sporadic prototypes of interactive medical simulation systems, improvements in hardware and software capabilities for providing natural interaction and graphical rendering, also in terms of VR, have led to an increasing adoption of such systems in medical practice. In fact, realism of 3D graphic and naturalness of interaction are key factors for medical simulation to be effective in a training context. VR systems for example, are increasingly focusing on improving the 'sense of presence' perceived by the user during the simulation. Natural interaction techniques can help to augment the immersivity of simulation by enabling users to interact with digital interfaces using gesture or voice input. As we described throughout the book, the increasing robustness of computer vision techniques allow to track user input using low-cost cameras, overcoming the problematic costs of dedicated tracking devices. Furthermore, CV algorithms applied to medical simulator

© The Author(s) 2017
81
A. Del Bimbo et al., *Natural Interaction in Medical Training*, SpringerBriefs in Human-Computer Interaction,
https://doi.org/10.1007/978-3-319-61036-8_5

systems can enable innovative functionalities. A precise user recognition based on visual appearance can be applied to a simulator in order to re-identity a trainee and track his progress or to associate the user with a specific role. In Chap. 3, we presented two effective methods based on computer vision to enable natural interaction in virtual simulations. The methods rely on low-cost RGB-D sensors to track user's hands pose and movement and to perform user re-identification.

Two prototypes of immersive virtual environment providing natural interaction were presented in Chap. 4. The systems were designed to train medical operators and professionals in the adoption and in the correct execution of medical procedures, i.e., the Basic Life Support and Defibrillation (BLSD) and the Surgical Safety Checklist (SSC). The adoption of these procedures in first aid emergencies and during surgical operations is essential in order to reduce mortality in victims and patients and to improve medical teams performance and learning. The main objective of the proposed systems has been therefore the design and implementation of a natural and immersive interfaces, sufficiently realistic and easy-to-use, to be actually adopted in medical education courses of study.

Immersive environments for medical simulation have been proven particularly effective in training complementary skills such as situation awareness, team dynamics, and adherence to procedures. One of the great advantage of virtual simulators is that they allow multiple repetitions at a low cost, allowing trainees to familiarize with complex healthcare procedures. Furthermore, virtual environments could be effectively adopted to reproduce extreme and dangerous situations, such as car accidents, large fires, or explosions with little cost and without putting doctors in any harm. In this context, simulation in the military field has been exploiting multi-user virtual environment for years to train army members in the battlefield. In the same way, a team of emergency medicine specialist could be trained with simulations of extreme scenarios using virtual reality and natural interaction.

We strongly believe that research in this field must be carried as a joint effort involving experts working in computer vision and pattern recognition, natural interaction, and medical personnel. We stress out the importance of involving trainers and trainees expert in different fields and with different roles not just as stakeholders but as active members co-designing the whole simulation. This is the only way to make sure developers pay attention to the important details in designing the simulation. This approach has been followed successfully in the two prototypes presented in Chap. 4.

Printed in the United States
By Bookmasters